The

Handbook

of

ALTERNATIVES

to

CHEMICAL MEDICINE

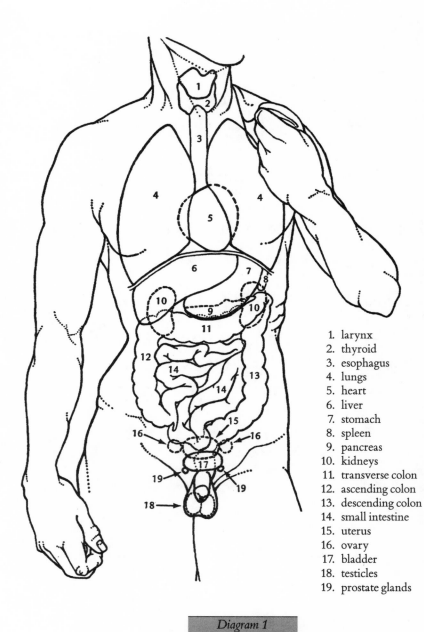

1. larynx
2. thyroid
3. esophagus
4. lungs
5. heart
6. liver
7. stomach
8. spleen
9. pancreas
10. kidneys
11. transverse colon
12. ascending colon
13. descending colon
14. small intestine
15. uterus
16. ovary
17. bladder
18. testicles
19. prostate glands

Diagram 1
INTERNAL ORGANS

The

Handbook

of

ALTERNATIVES

to

CHEMICAL MEDICINE

Mildred Jackson, N.D.

Terri K. Teague, N.D., D.C.

NEW WORLD LIBRARY

NOVATO, CALIFORNIA

New World Library
14 Pamaron Way
Novato, California 94949

Cover design by Meg Coughlin Design
Cover illustration by Jane Mjöelsness
Text illustrations by Martha Donovan-Anderson
Text layout and design by Aaron Kenedi

Library of Congress Cataloging-in-Publication Data

Jackson, Mildred.
The handbook of alternatives to chemical medicine / Mildred
Jackson, Terri K. Teague.
Previously published : Oakland, Calif. : Lawton-Teague
Includes bibliographical references and index.
ISBN 1-57731-059-4 (pbk.)
1. Naturopathy–Handbooks, manuals, etc. I. Teague, Terri.
II. Title
RZ440.J28 1997   97-11846
615.5–dc21   CIP

First printing, September 1997
Printed in Canada on acid-free paper
Distributed to the trade by Publishers Group West

10 9 8 7 6 5 4 3 2 1

For Mertianna, Eric, Jennifer, and Benjamin

Acknowledgments

 e *would like to thank all of the people* who have helped during the process of compiling this book. Many gave valuable advice, encouragement, and even advance financial support to an unpublished author and a tireless healer. If we have inadvertently left anyone out, we trust that this acknowledgment will serve as our thanks. A special thanks goes to Jim Lawton, Henry Poirot, Batyah Janowski, Adelaide Teague, Sylvia Sandifer, Michael Meyer, Nancy Kleban, Steve Brown, Barbara Apffel-Pierce, and Jerry Apffel-Pierce.

We would also like to thank Mrs. Morrie Blake, herbalist and cosmetologist, for her help since the first printing.

Table of Contents

$\mathscr{L}ist\ of\ \mathscr{D}iagrams$

Publisher's Preface

BY MARC ALLEN

ildred Jackson was a naturopathic doctor licensed to practice medicine using healing herbs and diet. She was legendary for her healing work and for her classes in the San Francisco Bay Area.

In the 1960s and early 1970s, she held a class every Thursday night in her little home in Albany, California, a quiet suburban community next to Berkeley. Her front room was filled with people, who sat on every chair and all over the floor as well, even spilling through the open double doors into her healing area. It was a quiet, attentive crowd, one that expected miracles to happen.

She would always begin her classes by reading from notebooks she had compiled over many years on the cures for illnesses and the powers of herbs and natural foods. Then she would answer questions — and heal everyone in the room with her answers. Often within her answers were stories of her past.

She never said how old she was, though she was certainly

well into her eighties, quite possibly in her nineties, when I met her in 1968. She said that at the age of seven she was told by a Native American woman that she had the gift of healing, and she studied healing from then on. She remembered everything our grandparents, and their parents and grandparents, knew about healing, but that our parents had forgotten, when they gave medical doctors, with their primary tools of drugs and surgery, responsibility for their health care. She often said that half her work was overcoming doctors' mistakes.

She also said she had trained to be a nurse, but was fired when she was asked to recite the Nurses' Creed. As I remember it, she said she had stood up, raised her right hand, and said, "Stand by your doctor when he's right, and expose him when he's wrong."

She charged twenty-five cents for her class — if you had it.

All day and all week long, she healed people in private sessions usually lasting about forty-five minutes each. She charged only five dollars for her sessions — again, if you had it — and in the 1970s finally raised her prices to seven dollars. She was a healer for the right reasons: compassion and love for people.

Terri Teague was one of her brightest, most enthusiastic students, and she became a naturopathic doctor as well. She worked with Mildred Jackson for countless hours over many months to condense her notes, which had been collected for sixty years or more, into a single volume. *The Handbook of Alternatives to Chemical Medicine* was the result of their labors — the result of a great many years of healing experience.

Here is some advice I remember from her classes, have used myself, or have recommended to people on many occasions:

* Begin your day with fruit juice. It cleanses your system. Wait awhile, then have cereal or some other good, natural breakfast.

* Drink lots of water. Mildred said, "Most people barely drink enough water to keep from dying of thirst."

* Eat lots of garlic. Mildred often said, "The list of what garlic cures is that long" — and she'd stretch out her hands to show that the list was at least three feet long.

And specific remedies:

* Cold remedy: Chicken soup — or hot vegetable soup for vegetarians (which she was) — with cayenne pepper or hot sauce. She said that cayenne pepper was very good for us in general.

* Internal infections, including bladder infections, kidney infections, and so on: Take a clove of garlic (not an entire bulb, like my aunt did), chop it up fine, put it in the bottom of a cup, and cover with a small amount of boiling water. Put a saucer over the top of the cup and let it sit all day. At night, just before going to bed, fill the cup with hot water — though not so hot you can't drink it comfortably — and drink it down, garlic pieces and all. You'll sleep very well, and the garlic will help the infection. She also recommended this for insomnia.

* Earache: Boil a clove of garlic until it is soft, let it cool a bit, and then gently place it in your ear. Hold it in place with a bit of

surgical tape. Sleep on it, and you'll feel better in the morning.

* Insomnia, nervousness, stress: Drink 2 cups of valerian root tea. (It smells like dirty socks, but doesn't taste too bad.) It has a wonderful sedative effect — every American should know about this tea. Camomile tea has the same effect, but is milder and tastes better.

* Pregnancy: During pregnancy, drink 2 cups raspberry leaf tea a day. It helps dilate the cervix during birth, making the baby's passage much easier. After the birth, drink 2 cups alfalfa tea a day. This helps remineralize the body, for a lot of essential minerals have been given to the baby. It makes the milk richer as well. Mix the tea with peppermint for better flavor.

* Hair Loss: Put $1/2$ ounce sage leaves and $1/2$ ounce rosemary leaves in a teapot. Cover with a pint of boiling water and let it steep for about 12 hours. Strain the herbs out and keep the remaining thick, black liquid in a jar in the refrigerator. Before you wash your hair in the morning, massage a generous amount of the liquid into your scalp, especially in areas where hair is thinning. Let your scalp absorb it for a few minutes, then wash as usual.

* Eyestrain, vision improvement: Sit relaxed with your eyes open. Then squeeze them shut tight for a moment, then open them wide. Look up, then down, moving your eyes as far as you comfortably can without moving your head. Repeat three to six times. Then look left, then right, as far as you can

without moving your head. Repeat three to six times. Then look up at the upper left corner of your eye, then the lower right corner, so you're looking diagonally across your field of vision. Repeat three to six times, then do it in the other direction, looking from the upper right corner to the lower left corner. Finish by circling your eyes round and round three to six times in as large a circle as you can comfortably make, then circle in the other direction. Mildred said that this exercise had helped improve her vision immensely.

These are only a few of the common, safe, simple remedies Mildred taught us. There are hundreds more in this book, the result of a very long lifetime of healing research and practice.

Mildred Jackson was a miracle worker, and it's not an exaggeration to say this. I'll never forget one of the first people I met in her classes. She was an attractive young woman, with striking clear brown eyes and perfect skin. She radiated good health. She told me she had leukemia. But before she underwent extensive radiation treatment, she chose to follow Mildred's advice first. Mildred told her to go somewhere quiet and restful in the country for three or four weeks, and to bring a good juicer with her. For two or three weeks, she followed Mildred's liquid diet (see the Cancer section in chapter 3). After that, Mildred put her on a healthy vegetarian diet, starting with vegetable soups. When the woman returned to the city and went back to her doctor, all signs of leukemia had vanished.

Mildred Jackson taught that there is no disease that can't be cured. We're designed to be strong and healthy and to live a long life. Eventually we age, but we can postpone that process for many, many years if we follow her advice.

Mildred lived to be, apparently, more than 100 years old (though I never knew how old she really was). She spent her long life healing thousands of people, and this book is her final contribution, making it possible for her healing work to continue, long after she has left us.

This edition of *The Handbook* is almost identical to the first edition printed more than twenty years ago. The only changes we made were to correct some typos and misspellings and to present remedies in a more consistent manner. We could have done more, but we wanted Mildred's voice to shine through. I hope we have succeeded.

Foreword

his is not your typical book on natural medicine. This book does not describe the benefits of presently popular nutritional supplements like DHEA, melatonin, or co-enzyme Q-10, nor does it mention newly popular herbal remedies such as gingko biloba, cat's claw, or kava.

What you will get from this book is Mildred Jackson's many decades of experience. Mildred Jackson lived, taught, and practiced into her nineties (she died in 1986). In this book, she and one of her students, Terri Teague, created a record of the remarkable variety of treatments that Mildred (and later, Terri) used successfully during years of practice.

What you will get from this book are tried and true remedies for common ailments. Many of the recommended treatments are unique to Dr. Jackson's experience and are not commonly described by other authors. These treatments will not always lead to rapid cures. In fact, many provide important nourishment that then enables the body to heal itself — in its own time. The simple beauty of the recommendations made in this book is their safety.

Another special benefit of this book is the variety of recommended treatments the authors provide. If or when one treatment doesn't work adequately, another can be tried.

This book does not provide commentary on, or critique of, conventional medicine. The authors felt it unnecessary to attack conventional medicine; they found it simply more appropriate to give people options and let them choose for themselves.

This book does not try to give scientific evidence or a rationale for the efficacy of any treatment. Instead, the authors have written about what works for them.

Drs. Jackson and Teague wrote this book before many of the relatively new scientific studies began to confirm the preventive and therapeutic value of "nutriceuticals" (healing nutrients in food) and "phytochemicals" (healing nutrients in plants). Since *The Handbook of Alternatives to Chemical Medicine* was first published, a growing body of evidence has accumulated to verify the rationale and effectiveness of many treatments the authors recommended.

Don't just read this book; use this book...just for the health of it.

— Dana Ullman, M.P.H.
Berkeley, California

Author of *The Consumer's Guide to Homeopathy, Homeopathic Medicines for Children and Infants,* and coauthor of *Everybody's Guide to Homeopathic Medicine.*

CHAPTER 1

Guidelines to Health

properly functioning body is no accident. It is the result of consumption of the proper foods, adequate exercise, and regulation of your environment. All organs of the body are interrelated, and a malfunction in one will create disturbances in all the others. You must become familiar with your body and its needs. Each one mends at a different rate because we are each physically and chemically unique, and requirements for nourishment, exercise, and environment vary from individual to individual.

It is important to remember that the harmony of health, and not the disharmony of disease, is the normal state of the body. Achievement of this normal state is made difficult by our fast-paced society, the primary byproducts of which are tension, confusion, and pressure. Yet in the face of these distractions, each of us bears the responsibility for our health and that of our children and charges. It is comforting to know that there is a simple and inexpensive alternative to high blood pressure and high medical and pharmaceutical bills.

Eating and Drinking

Eating is the favorite pastime of many, and the downfall of some. Nutritional imbalances play a large part in the originating causes of disease. Devitalized foods, such as cane sugar, white flour, and foods with chemical additives, cannot supply the proper amounts of amino acids that nourish every cell in the body. Here are some informative hints on how to enjoy your food and derive more benefit from it by allowing your body to function at its best during the processes of digestion and assimilation.

CHEWING

When you sit down to eat, make sure that you have plenty of time to relax and enjoy your meal — and make sure that you are hungry! If you have only five minutes to "grab a bite to eat," skip the meal and sip a glass of juice or water instead. Wait until you have plenty of time to eat without swallowing your food whole. Gulping food or liquids does a tremendous disservice to your stomach and may result in headaches, stomachaches, gas, and constipation. The hurried eater also loses part of the benefits of the vitamins and minerals in food because the digestive system is unable to continue functioning properly when the first step, mastication, is slighted. Saliva, secreted by the salivary glands, breaks down the starches and sugars in food and prepares them for the gastric juices in the stomach. Hastily eaten food misses the primary digestive process that depends upon thorough chewing and grinding in the mouth.

DRINKING

Drinking with meals can cause indigestion and gas. Food misses the salivary treatment when it is washed down with a drink. The food, then, must be broken down in the stomach, where it collides with the liquid and creates chaos. It is best to drink something at least half an hour before meals, and preferably an hour. This rule applies to water, wine, milk, and all other liquids. The same time interval should be observed when drinking after a meal as well. Chronic stomach problems will often clear up within a week if this routine is observed faithfully.

You are wasting your body's energy if you gulp your food or liquids. Gulped liquids rush through the system, and your body does not have time to replenish and cleanse its cells. Sipping gives you the full benefit of the drink. Ideally, it should take you an hour to sip 8 ounces of water, and your body needs at least 24 ounces of water a day in addition to juices and herbal teas. When you drink the necessary amount of liquids, your body feels hungry less often because your cells are no longer screaming for nourishment. Two-thirds of the body is made up of water. The body uses water to flush out used dead cells, toxins, and other wastes. All the body organs will suffer if proper amounts of water are not supplied. The kidneys, particularly, need water to function properly, and when toxins cannot be flushed out by the kidneys, lower back pain can result.

Ice-cold drinks can retard digestion and shock the stomach, especially after exercise. So try to drink them at room temperature instead.

EATING FRUITS AND VEGETABLES

Fruits and vegetables eaten together or fruits eaten with other fruits may wipe out the nutritional benefits of both! Each fruit contains a different type of acid, and when one fruit is combined with another, the stomach becomes a battleground of acids. Consequently, fewer vitamins and minerals can be assimilated effectively by the system. Each day choose one type of fruit and eat as much of it as you like, but wait until the next day to have another. If you have little bumps on the ends of your fingers, you may have been eating combinations of fruits. The bumps — indicating a slightly irritated skin condition — are due to the concentration of acids in conflict.

Fruits should never be eaten with vegetables. Vegetables may be eaten in all combinations without loss of benefits, but not within an hour of eating fruit. Occasionally, you may wish to cheat and enjoy orange sauce on duck with asparagus, but fruit salads with dinner can create havoc in your stomach.

OVEREATING

Overeating creates problems throughout the system. A great many Americans suffer from distended colons, one of the results of overindulgence. Many of us, particularly in this country, feel a need to overeat because of the quality of the foods that we consume. When we eat devitalized foods, the body is left with a feeling of dissatisfaction and sends signals to the brain that we are still hungry. When the proper foods are eaten, after a certain period of adjustment the body will feel satisfied on far less. If you will eat only what you need, your body will not have to work so hard and you will be freer of headaches and feelings of sluggishness.

SAVING YOUR STOMACH IN THE MORNING

The first thing your body needs in the morning is fruit or fruit juice. The remains of last night's dinner may not yet be out of the stomach, and the juice will help to clean out this food and prepare your stomach for today's food. Coffee and other strong acidic substances, when taken first thing in the morning, meet the undigested food and create an explosion of gases. Fresh fruit or fruit juice stimulates the digestive process and gives your body a good start on the day. Orange juice may contain too much fruit sugar and tomato juice too much acid, but any type of juice you prefer is fine. You may eat or drink any type of fruit or fruit juice and have as much of it as you like, but wait at least half an hour before eating anything else. If you start the day this way, you will find yourself more cheerful in the mornings and ready to tackle the day's activities.

Exercise

Physical exercise facilitates proper digestion. Lack of physical exercise causes clogging in both the digestive tract and the glandular system. Exercise should be part of your daily routine and need not be strenuous or inconvenient. Swimming, dancing, walking, and simply stretching stimulate the body and help to relax tensions.

Thinking

Worry and fear are major causes of disease, and psychosomatic illnesses are as painful and uncomfortable as organic ones are. In fact, anxiety over disease can not only make you think you are ill, but can actually make you ill! Many parents inadvertently encourage illness in their children by overreacting. If you tell your child that he or she is going to catch a cold, you are encouraging disease rather than health. On the other hand, parents can promote health and facilitate healing by encouraging their children to be well.

Many of us worry about major misfortune and, in doing so, create stresses that deplete our reserves of vitamins and minerals. If your body is allowed to function properly, you will not only be less likely to think about being ill, but your natural resistance will protect you from sickness. Alfalfa or red clover, taken daily in tablet or tea form, will restore a high level of resistance. Colds, flu, and even children's diseases such as mumps and measles can be avoided if the body resistance is kept high.

Anger, dissatisfaction, and negativity inhibit the body's ability to function naturally and create an atmosphere within the body conducive to disease. Hateful thoughts do enormous harm to your system. Worry, anger, or hate can produce up to one pint of acid per minute in the body. So prolonged negative thoughts create a tremendous chemical imbalance in the body. Approaching problems with a calm and collected attitude will do wonders for your physical and mental well-being.

CHAPTER 2

Guidelines to Preparation

other Nature *has provided us with a natural remedy* for almost any disease or malfunction, but you will benefit far more from her provisions if you know how to properly prepare your treatments. For the best results, follow the instructions given with each treatment, at least until you are familiar with its effects and results. Do not use herbal treatments while taking a chemical medication.

Because each of us is unique, some of us will respond better to one treatment and some to another. There are often many treatments given for one disease, and you may use the one you prefer. I have marked the remedies that I find most effective with a *.

Do not expect an ailment of 15 years to disappear overnight. On the other hand, once an ailment has been effectively treated herbally, there is little chance of recurrence as the herbs stimulate the body's production and protection mechanisms.

Herbs can be grown both indoors and outdoors, or may

be purchased. Some are listed in the appendices. It is always best to use organically grown herbs. Herbs keep best in tightly sealed glass or ceramic containers and should not be exposed to direct sunlight or drastic temperature changes. Herbs that are grown, harvested, and stored properly are more potent. Herbs also lose strength with age and should be discarded after 12–15 months, depending on the herb.

When preparing a treatment, make sure that you are using the correct part of the plant. The flowers, stems, leaves, and roots of a plant may each have different properties, and when this is so, specific parts of the plant have been designated as the most useful. Herbal treatments are quite safe if directions are followed. Excesses, however, may reduce the efficiency of the treatment.

Do not use aluminum utensils, pots, pans, or storage containers for any food-related use. When water or food comes in contact with aluminum, it undergoes a chemical change and picks up tiny particles of aluminum that accumulate in the liver, spleen, and kidneys. Needless to say, aluminum should never be used, not even for your pet's dishes.

Use only organically grown fruits and vegetables, especially when peels are used. Pesticides do not belong in healing remedies.

Teas

Herbs are usually taken in teas prepared in the following way: Place the herb in a ceramic or glass container, pour boiling water over it, and allow it to steep. Generally teas are made with a ratio of 1 teaspoon herb to 1 cup boiling water. Unless a recipe specifically instructs, do not boil the herb with the water because that can destroy the beneficial characteristics of the herb. Also, as a general rule, do not combine more than three herbs. If a particular tea seems bitter, you may add honey, but don't add sugar because it lessens the useful properties of the herb and also depletes the body's reserves of vitamins and minerals. Pure honey, on the other hand, is a natural sweetener that also contains valuable nutrients.

Poultices

Poultices are useful for sprains, ruptures, tension and swelling, for drawing out infections, and for drawing together cuts and broken bones. Poultices are most effective when made of fresh, organically grown fruits, vegetables, or leaves that are grated, chopped, or crushed as directed. The herb is then wrapped in a clean, well-woven, nonirritating fabric such as muslin or cotton, and applied externally. In some cases, such as whiplash, it is best to use a cloth of pure silk or silk mixture, such as a scarf. As a last resort, paper towels may be used for poultices that are to be applied for no more than 10 or 15 minutes. Colored or recycled paper towels, however, may contain impurities that will interfere with the healing process.

Poultices should be slightly damp and may be covered with a plastic bag to hold in the moisture. The poultice should be changed when dry, or every 3 to 5 hours depending upon the severity of the condition. Each time the poultice is changed, replace the cloth with a clean one.

If fresh herbs are not available, use dried herbs and pour boiling water over them to soften before placing inside the cloth.

Comfrey poultices are the most frequently used and are very simply made. Cut a piece of cloth twice as large as the area you wish to cover and use a freshly picked comfrey leaf. Wash the leaf in cool water and crush it in your hand. Spread the leaf on one side of the cloth, fold over the other half and apply to the affected part of the body (see Diagram 2). Do not place the comfrey leaf directly against the skin because the leaf fuzz will irritate the skin. If the poultice is made with comfrey root or dried leaves, pour boiling water over the herb to soften and use the strained root or leaves in the poultice. Drink the resulting tea.

Diagram 2

HOW TO PREPARE
A POULTICE

Your Home Medicine Chest

Your medicine cabinet need only contain the following items: garlic, alfalfa, comfrey, aloe vera, and lemon. With these articles you can effectively treat almost every disease or condition. Garlic has been nicknamed the "body cleanser" because it can clean the entire blood system in less than an hour. Garlic also contains many nutrients. Alfalfa helps oxidize the blood, fight infection, and build up the body's resistance to disease. Comfrey, also known as knitbone, can be used for pulling cuts together, relieving swelling, dissolving internal growths, and drawing broken bones back into place. Comfrey has also been used to repair ruptured hernias in less than 2 weeks. Aloe vera is a form of cactus with wonderful medicinal properties. It soothes burns, relieves toothaches, helps heal cuts and bruises, and can be used for chapped lips and rough skin. Lemon juice is the most antiseptic liquid known to man, more effective than rubbing alcohol or peroxide. Lemon juice soothes itchy bites and skin rashes, and when taken internally with water helps cleanse, tone, and relax the entire system. In addition, 1 drop of lemon juice in an eye cup of warm water is a refreshing bath for the eyes.

With these herbs on hand, you are well prepared to deal effectively with any emergency.

CHAPTER 3

Remedies

ackache

Many people suffer from back pain. If your pelvis or any vertebrae is out of alignment, you should see a naturopath, osteopath, or chiropractor. He or she will be able to realign your vertebrae or reposition your pelvis. Occasionally, a negative mental state will cause pain in the back. "Burden-bearing thoughts" can help create backache. If this is the case, a positive outlook should bring relief.

The lower back, or lumbar region, can become painful if you are not drinking enough water. If you do not take the time to drink sufficient fluids, the kidneys will not function properly and the resultant toxicity can cause pain. Make sure you are drinking enough fluids (sipping, not gulping!). Sip at least three 8-ounce glasses of water per day in addition to herbal teas and juices.

Massage the feet along the instep to help increase the circulation in the back and relax tension that may be concentrated there.

Dried Boston ivy is helpful for backaches. Use in tea; make with 1 ounce herb in 1 quart boiling water and allow to cool. Drink 2–3 cups per day for 6 weeks to 2 months.

A poultice of bacon fat applied externally to the back will help to draw out pain.

SCIATICA
The sciatic nerve runs from the heel of the foot up the legs and through the body. Massaging the back of the heel and up the entire leg can help to relieve the pain of sciatica.

Jasmine oil will help to soothe sciatic pain, and the bark may be made into a tea. Use 1/2 teaspoon bark to 1 cup boiling water and steep for 3–5 minutes. Drink 1–2 cups per day as needed.

Vitamin D, taken with calcium and magnesium, will be assimilated properly by the body and help to ease sciatic pain.

To treat sciatica, combine 1/2 cup darnel, 1/2 teaspoon honey, and 1 1/2 cups distilled water. Steep several minutes, strain, and sip slowly, 1/2 cup at a time, during the day.

Rue is a good treatment for sciatic pain. Make a tea using 1 teaspoon rue to 1 cup boiling water. Steep 5 minutes, strain, and drink 2–3 cups daily or when needed.

Brain

All diseases of the brain, from insomnia to psychosis, can be treated with herbs, counseling, and a healthy mental attitude. Many severe emotional disturbances originate from prolonged vitamin and mineral deficiencies. The brain requires plenty of lecithin, calcium, phosphorous, and vitamins B and C, but without enough of *any* nutrient, the brain will suffer. Adequate daily exercise and a cheerful disposition will help to revitalize the brain and keep it healthy.

ALL BRAIN MALFUNCTIONS
Lecithin is needed by the brain in order to function properly, and it is recommended for all brain disorders. One tablespoon daily in liquid, granule, or capsule form is sufficient. Lecithin is found in fertile eggs, soy products, and in small amounts in all vegetables that have been vine ripened.

Phosphorus is essential to proper brain functioning. It is found in caraway seeds, apples and apple seeds, marigold, chipweed, and horsetail herb. One or more of these herbs should be taken in tea or eaten daily.

BRAIN DAMAGE
Masterwort herb will stimulate the activity of the organs and help to reduce paralysis caused by hemorrhaging of the brain or spinal column. Use 1 ounce root to 1 pint boiling water and drink ½ cup three times a day.

Black walnut hull tea will help to restore damaged cells in the brain. Use 1 teaspoon hulls to 1 cup boiling water and steep for 10–15 minutes. Slowly sip 3 cups per day.

Mongolism may be caused by improper assimilation of vitamins and minerals by the mother during pregnancy. The child should be given vitamins B, C, and E daily in food and in supplemental form to help stimulate normal growth.

Sage tea is an excellent treatment for mental retardation because it will increase circulation to the brain and feed the cortex. Use 1 teaspoon sage to 1 cup boiling water and drink 3–5 cups per day for 6 months to 1 year. Improvement should be obvious and treatment should be continued as needed.

BRAIN TONICS

*Sage tea helps to revitalize the brain and improve concentration. Sage supplies oxygen to the cortex of the brain. Use 1 teaspoon sage to 1 cup boiling water and steep 3–5 minutes. Drink freely.

Mugwort and rosemary help to relieve mental fatigue and forgetfulness. Use 1 teaspoon combined herbs to 1 cup boiling water. Drink 3 cups per day.

Yerba mate will help stimulate the intellect and the body and tone the intestinal tract. Yerba mate is high in vitamin C, magnesium, silica, and phosphates, which feed the system. Use 1 teaspoon yerba mate to 1 cup boiling water and drink 3 cups per day.

Camomile stimulates the brain and helps to dispel weariness. Use 1 teaspoon flowers to 1 cup boiling water and drink freely.

Dissolve $1/2$ teaspoon barley in 2 cups boiling water, steep for 10 minutes, and take daily to help strengthen the brain.

Blend the following ingredients for 5 minutes and sip slowly. This mixture contains iron, vitamin C, and many other nutrients that act as a tonic for the brain cells.

> *$1/2$ cup apricot juice*
> *1 teaspoon lemon juice*
> *1 pinch kelp*
> *1 fertile egg yolk*
> *1 $1/2$ cups soy or goat milk*

Dolomite (calcium and magnesium) aids the memory processes. Take 2–4 tablets per day. Each tablet contains approximately 125 mg. calcium and 75 mg. magnesium.

ALCOHOLISM

Alcohol destroys calcium, magnesium, iron, and all vitamins, particularly vitamins B and D. Raw honey will supply some of these nutrients; also use vitamin and mineral supplements.

Delirium tremens (DTs) should be treated with bugle. This herb is a mild sedative and will help to control hallucinations. Use 1 teaspoon powdered bugle to 1 cup boiling water and drink 3 cups per day, or take 5 grains daily in capsule form.

Angelica root or leaves will help to destroy the desire for alcohol. Use 1 teaspoon root or leaves to 1 cup boiling water. Drink 3 cups per day.

AUTISM

Autistic children should be given plenty of fresh, raw vegetables and fruits and fresh juices. Do not let the autistic child eat any processed foods or foods containing chemical additives or colorings. The autistic child may be calmed by placing the hand on the back of the child's neck which helps to reorient the child to surrounding energy. Sage tea will help to strengthen the brain and relax fear and tension. Use 1 teaspoon sage to 1 cup boiling water and sweeten with honey. Drink 3 or more cups per day.

DEPRESSION AND RESTLESSNESS

Chronic melancholy or depression may be caused by deficiencies of vitamins C and E. Take these vitamins daily.

If the spleen is not producing enough red blood cells, the subsequent lack of oxygen can cause depression. To stimulate the spleen, place the following herbs in a burlap sack. Pour two quarts boiling water onto the herbs and allow the mixture to steep for 24 hours. Then add 4 ounces natural honey to the strained liquid and drink 1–2 cups when depressed.

> *4 ounces hawthorne*
> *1 ounce cardamom*
> *1 ounce saffron*
> *¹/₂ cup each balm and red sage*

Balm and ground ivy will help restore the spirits. Make a tea using 1 teaspoon combined herbs to 1 cup boiling water. Sweeten with honey to taste and drink when needed. Or, make balm leaf tea using $^1/_2$ teaspoon leaves to 1 cup boiling water. Drink 3 cups per day.

Mayflowers will help to relieve nervous depression, restlessness, and general pessimism. Use 1 teaspoon fresh plant to 1 cup boiling water. Take 2 cups per day.

Fit root helps relieve restlessness and spasms. Use 1 teaspoon powdered root to 1 cup boiling water. Steep for 20 minutes and drink 2 cups per day.

Dodder is a good herb for the treatment of hypochondria. Make a tea using 1 teaspoon herb to 1 cup boiling water. Drink 3 cups per day until condition clears.

Myrrh, when burned as incense, will clear away negative energy. When taken as a tea, it will lift the spirits. Use $^1/_2$ teaspoon powdered herb to 1 cup boiling water and drink 1–2 cups per day.

Passion flower is a good treatment for hysteria and will relax nervous tension. Use 1 teaspoon herb to 1 cup boiling water and drink 2 cups per day.

Peppermint tea will help to relieve moodiness and relax the heart. Use 1 heaping teaspoon leaves in 1 cup boiling water. Drink freely.

A tea made of peppermint, catnip, rue, and wood betony will help to clear obstructions in the system and relieve dizziness. Use 1 teaspoon combined herbs to 1 cup boiling water. Drink early in the day.

EPILEPSY

Epilepsy is caused by toxemia, or excess toxins in the system. This disease is characterized by nervous spasms and convulsions called seizures. When the body goes into convulsions, the seizure has already occurred within the brain. The body reacts to the seizure with a rush of adrenalin, which, added to the excess toxins already in the blood, causes the nervous reaction of convulsion. At this point, the more blood you can divert to the brain to ease the shock and eliminate the excess adrenalin, the sooner the convulsions will cease. To help control seizures, place a belt around each leg between the knee and thigh and pull it tight (see Diagram 3). Leave the belts in place for 1–2 minutes and release. This procedure will divert the blood flow to the upper part of the body, particularly the brain, and help to shorten the muscle spasms. Another way to help reduce a seizure is to step firmly on the patient's little finger of either hand. During all seizures take care to protect the patient from harm. After a seizure have the patient breathe fresh air and move around to stimulate circulation and minimize the aftereffects of the seizure.

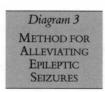

Diagram 3
METHOD FOR ALLEVIATING EPILEPTIC SEIZURES

Epileptics should be sure they are getting plenty of B-complex vitamins and that they are not deficient in zinc. Dolomite (calcium and magnesium) and lecithin are also helpful when treating epilepsy.

Dittany is one of the best treatments for epilepsy. When taken daily for 6 months or more, dittany has been known to control seizures and gradually help stop them altogether. Use 1 teaspoon herb in 1 cup boiling water and steep for 5 minutes. Take 1 tablespoon tea 3 times a day. During this treatment abstain from all meats except fish or poultry and take no chemicals into the body. Continue treatment whether seizures occur or not.

Cinquefoil is a good treatment for epilepsy and other diseases of the brain. Cinquefoil tea helps to remove poisons and congestion from any part of the body. Use 1 teaspoon root to 1 cup boiling water and take 2–3 cups per day. Continue for 6 months to 2 years or until all symptoms are gone.

Snakeroot is a good treatment for epilepsy because it is an antispasmodic herb. Use ¹⁄₂ ounce powdered plant to 1 pint boiling water. Take 3 cups per day.

Use 1 teaspoon valerian herb to 1 cup boiling water for epilepsy. Drink 2–3 cups per day.

Basswood is a good treatment for epilepsy. Use 1 teaspoon in 1 cup boiling water, steep 3–5 minutes, and take ¹⁄₂ cup 4 times a day.

Calamint will promote recovery from all brain ailments. Use 1 teaspoon leaves and flowers in 1 cup boiling water and drink 2 cups per day.

INSANITY

American mandrake sap can be used to treat all forms of insanity. Take 1/2 teaspoon fresh sap daily or use 1 teaspoon mandrake plant in 1 cup boiling water to make a tea. Drink 3 cups daily. Continue as necessary.

Holly seeds help strengthen the memory and are a useful treatment for all types of insanity. Make a tea using 1/2 teaspoon seeds to 1 cup boiling water. Drink 3 cups per day.

Make a tea using 1 teaspoon powdered vervain plant to 1 cup boiling water. Drink 1 cup every hour to treat all types of insanity.

Snakeroot tea is a good treatment for all mental disorders. This bitter herb will help cleanse the system of poisons. Use 1 teaspoon root to 1 cup boiling water or take an equivalent amount in capsule form.

Carrot seed tea helps in the treatment of all mental disorders by relaxing tension. Use 1 teaspoon seeds in 1 cup boiling water. Drink 2–3 cups per day.

INSOMNIA

*For chronic sleeplessness, chop 1 clove garlic and place in a glass with just enough water to cover. Place a lid on the glass and allow the mixture to stand all day. Just before bedtime fill the glass with water, as warm as you can drink, and sip slowly. Repeat this treatment daily for 10 days to 2 weeks.

Sleeplessness is caused by an inability to relax. To promote relaxation, lie on the floor and slowly tense each part of the body beginning with the toes and working up the legs, torso, arms, neck, and head. When the entire body is tense, release the tension altogether. This helps the body release tension.

Cucumbers are good for calming tension because they contain hormones and plenty of calcium.

Leaving salt out of the evening meal helps to promote sleep. The salt acts as a stimulant to the system. Replacing the salt needs with dulse also gives a relaxing boost to the thyroid and glandular system.

Strawberry leaves make a tasty, relaxing tea. Use 1 teaspoon leaves to 1 cup boiling water. Sip warm tea slowly before bed.

Camomile tea helps to calm the nerves, revitalize the body, and stimulate the circulation in the hands and feet. Use 1 teaspoon herb to 1 cup boiling water. Steep for 10 minutes, strain, and drink before retiring.

Rosehips tea, taken before bed, helps facilitate sound sleep. The high amount of vitamin C in rosehips helps calm and soothe the nerves. Use 1 teaspoon hips to 1 cup boiling water, steep for 10 minutes, strain, and drink before bed.

A small amount of oil of cloves, taken with honey, helps to relax tense muscles.

One or two tablets of calcium (5–7 grains) in a glass of warm milk before bed will help you get to sleep.

One teaspoon nutmeg taken in juice or milk before bed will help to relax tension and promote sleep.

To aid sleep, combine 4 tablespoons each skullcap, nerve root, and mint flowers with 1 quart water and boil mixture down to 1 pint. Drink 2 cups per day.

Carob leaf tea is relaxing to the entire nervous system. Use 1 teaspoon leaves to 1 cup boiling water and steep for 5 minutes. Take as needed for nervousness.

Lemon leaves, simmered for 20 minutes in 1 $^1/_2$ cups water, help relax tension and aid sleep. Drink before bed.

Raw or juiced celery is good for all types of nervousness and will help relax tension. Take daily when needed.

Make a tea with lungwort, using 1 teaspoon leaves to 1 cup boiling water. Take twice a day to help promote relaxation.

English lettuce helps to relax the nerves and promote sleep. It can be eaten raw in salads or juiced.

Hops flower tea will help relax the spinal column. Use 1 teaspoon flowers to 1 cup boiling water and drink several cups a day or when needed. Also, use a pillow stuffed with hops flowers to relax the body and promote sleep.

MANIC DEPRESSION

Manic episodes may be controlled by giving the patient grapefruit sections with raw honey. This treatment will calm the nerves and supply the body with vitamin C and pantothenic acid. Manic-depressives should follow the diet recommended for schizophrenia, adding plenty of fresh vegetable juices.

The remedies previously recommended in the Depression and Restlessness section will also be helpful for manic depression.

SCHIZOPHRENIA

Drink several glasses a day of carrot juice mixed with sage to help control schizophrenia. This combination will help to reduce the nervous tension and strengthen the brain. To keep the system clean and functional, eat only raw vegetables, fish or poultry, and plenty of fruit. Do not eat red meat, sugar products, or processed foods.

SENILITY

Senility is not an incurable or unavoidable disease. The symptoms of senility are caused by vitamin and mineral deficiencies in the system. As the body ages, more calcium is needed to keep the bones firm, the nervous system requires more vitamin C, and more potassium is needed to maintain muscle strength. An absence of any vitamin or mineral will inhibit proper functioning of an aging system. Be sure a well-balanced diet is followed. See the appendices for lists of foods high in these nutrients.

Sage tea will help stop trembling of the limbs. Use 1 teaspoon herb to 1 cup boiling water and drink freely. This tea will also help strengthen the brain and memory.

SIMPLE TENSION AND NERVOUSNESS

A daily warm bath, followed by a cool bath of salt water, helps relax the nervous system. Swimming in the ocean is always beneficial.

Dill strengthens the brain and calms tension in the stomach. Use 1 teaspoon herb to 1 cup boiling water. Drink several cups per day.

Juniper berries tone the nerves and strengthen the brain. Make a tea using 1 teaspoon berries to 1 cup boiling water. Steep for 5 minutes, strain, and drink 2–3 cups per day.

Chia seeds help to calm the nerves. They may be made into tea or added to salads or cooking. To make in tea, use 1 teaspoon seeds to 1 cup boiling water. Drink 2–3 cups per day.

Restlessness may be caused by a need for calcium, magnesium, and vitamin D. Turnips are a good source of these nutrients.

Basil is good for the nerves. Use 1 teaspoon in 1 pint water. Sip slowly during the day to calm tension.

Skullcap is a nervine and is also beneficial for the heart. It helps relax tension and promote sleep. Use 1 teaspoon in 1 cup boiling water, steep 3–5 minutes, and drink when needed.

Valerian helps calm the nerves. Use 1 teaspoon herb to 1 cup boiling water and drink 2–3 cups per day.

Lemon juice and water sipped throughout the day will help tone the system and calm the nerves. Use the juice of one lemon in 8 ounces water. Repeat up to six times.

Parsley tea is a mild sedative and contains nourishing vitamins and minerals. Use 1 teaspoon parsley to 1 cup boiling water, or eat the fresh herb. Take as often as needed.

Before sleeping, drink a mixture of $1/2$ cup orange juice, $1/2$ cup pineapple juice, and $1/4$ cup lemon juice. The combination will help to relax the body for sleep.

Garlic and onions are both powerful sedatives that soothe the brain. Use separately or mix together in tea and drink several cups per day.

Cancer, Tumors, and Cysts

Cancer is one of the most dreaded diseases, but it can be controlled and even eliminated with the proper mental attitude and diet. Most cancers begin in the same way: an organ or section of the circulatory system becomes clogged with impurities that stagnate and begin to reproduce. To alleviate the condition, the blood stream and all the organs must be thoroughly cleansed. If you are told you have cancer, immediately exclude from the diet all protein foods such as meat, eggs, beans, lentils, and cheese. This will "starve" the reproducing cells. Eat only raw fruits, vegetables, and juices; these foods will cleanse the system and allow the body to fight the cancer. If the treatment is to be successful, the entire system must be kept free of all obstructions and the blood stream must be kept pure.

Poultices should be used directly over the affected external area and over the diseased internal area. During all stages of treatment, drink only distilled water and eat plenty of roughage foods. A diet consisting of raw fruit for one meal, raw vegetables for the next, then fruit again, etc., is the best to follow. Other than fruits, vegetables, and juices, eat one slice of sourdough bread each day. Continue the diet until all growths are gone and the body has returned to functioning properly.

INTERNAL AND EXTERNAL CANCERS
*Make the following juices fresh daily and, in addition, drink at least three 8-ounce glasses of water. Eat no other foods. This diet will supply the body with all the nutrients needed, but will not support cancerous growths.

On day 1, drink 10 ounces carrot juice and 6 ounces spinach juice.

On day 2, drink 3 ounces spinach juice, 2 ounces parsley juice, 4 ounces celery juice, and 7 ounces carrot juice.

On day 3, drink 3 ounces each of beet and cucumber

juice, and 10 ounces carrot juice.

On day 4, drink 2 ounces coconut juice, 3 ounces beet juice, and 11 ounces carrot juice.

On day 5, drink 1 pint spinach juice.

On day 6, drink 2 ounces parsley juice, 5 ounces celery juice, and 9 ounces carrot juice.

On day 7, drink 12 ounces carrot juice and 4 ounces parsley juice.

On day 8, start the diet over again with day 1 and continue in sequence until condition is completely cleared.

Watercress helps supply vitamins and nutrients to the system and helps to clear cancerous growths. Eat in salad or drink juice daily.

Horsetail herb is a good treatment for both internal and external cancers. Use 2 large handfuls in 1 quart boiling water, steep for 10 minutes, and strain. Add honey, if needed, and drink 4–5 cups daily.

Oatstraw helps rebuild the minerals in the system. A cloth soaked in oatstraw tea and placed on the skin will help to stop decay and control engorgement. Make a tea using 2 large handfuls oatstraw to 1 quart boiling water. Let steep for 10 minutes, strain, and apply externally. In addition, drink 4–5 cups per day.

To reduce the offensive odor of cancerous decay, use powdered charcoal and yeast in a poultice over the affected areas. Change the poultice often and burn the cloth and residue.

Grated raw carrot, made into a poultice, will help soothe inflammation and reduce odor. Cooked, raw, and juiced carrots are beneficial for all types of cancer because of the nutrients they contain. If carrots are cooked, be sure to drink the liquid in which they cook.

Grapes help to control cancer because they contain cell salts that nourish the blood system. A diet of nothing but grapes may be eaten for 3 months. Take care to drink only distilled water, at least 1 cup per hour. When using the grape diet, eat the seeds, skin, and meat of the grape.

Comfrey leaves in a poultice will help control cancerous growths and, when combined with comfrey tea, will help to clean out the system. Drink 5 or more cups of tea per day and change the poultices at least three times a day.

To help heal cancerous growths, use $1/2$ pound red clover to 1 pint water. Simmer the mixture until it is reduced to a syrup. Watch carefully to prevent burning. Spread syrup onto a cloth and apply daily. Repeat until completely cleared.

A poultice of crushed, fresh cranberries will raise pustules on the cancerous skin. The "blistering" is the cancerous tissue being drawn out of the body. Change the poultice at least three times a day, gently wipe the area with a clean, sterile cloth, and reapply poultice. Continue until pustules no longer appear.

Crush fresh blue or white violet leaves and use in a poultice to help draw out cancerous growths. Also, make a tea of the leaves. Use 1 teaspoon leaves to 1 cup boiling water and drink 3–5 cups per day.

Sarcoidosis, a form of cancer of the lungs, may be treated by using the cranberry poultice regimen along with daily breathing exercises. Fill the lungs with air from the abdomen up through the chest. This will help to strengthen the lungs and ensure an adequate supply of oxygen.

BRAIN TUMORS

Tumors in the brain may be drawn out by placing a poultice of fresh grape juice at the nape of the neck. This poultice should be changed when dry and treatment should be continued until the growth is gone. Comfrey tea and plenty of raw juices will help to facilitate this process.

CYSTS

Cysts anywhere in the body may be treated with comfrey tea. This tea should be drunk five or more times a day to help the healing process, and a comfrey poultice should be placed on the skin outside the affected area.

The juice diet given at the beginning of this section is another helpful way to treat cysts of the internal organs. Follow the diet for at least 10 days to ensure that the cysts are dissolved.

Dolomite and garlic pearlies (garlic oil in capsules) are helpful for dissolving cysts. Take in tablet form or eat in foods.

LEUKEMIA

Leukemia is a form of cancer that destroys the marrow of the bones. The same diets may be used and cranberry juice should be added. The liver, spleen, and pancreas must be kept clean and functional so that new blood cells can be produced as quickly as they are needed.

Chronic and Degenerative Diseases

Most degenerative diseases, including multiple sclerosis (MS), muscular dystrophy, and palsy, are caused by a form of malnutrition that results from a continuous diet of devitalized and processed foods. Vitamin deficiencies from this type of diet will result in the deterioration of the myelin sheath that covers and protects the nerves. This breakdown of myelin causes a loss of resistance to infection, muscular spasms, and a gradual loss of control over the entire muscle system. Fatty acids contain vitamin F and this deficiency, coupled with deficiencies of vitamins B, C, and E as well as dolomite, will eventually cripple the body. To treat these diseases, the first step is to completely eliminate from the diet all processed foods, liquids, and sugars. Brown rice contains many nourishing minerals and vitamins that can help rebuild the nervous system. The following remedies are also helpful.

DROPSY (EDEMA)

Dropsy is the condition of excessive water retention in the body. If not remedied, an extreme case of dropsy can literally drown the patient. Dropsy indicates that the kidneys, pancreas, and liver are all malfunctioning. The sections dealing with diseases of these organs will give further information on specific treatments. Here are some general remedies for dropsy.

For Bright's disease and dropsy, take queen-of-the-meadow root tea. Use 1 teaspoon root to 1 cup boiling water, steep for 10 minutes, and drink ¹/₂ cup three times per day.

The inner bark of the white ash is a good treatment for dropsy. Steep 1 teaspoon in 1 cup boiling water for 30 minutes. Strain and drink ¹/₂ glass four to five times a day.

Juniper berries help the body to eliminate excess fluids. Use 5–7 berries to 1 pint boiling water. Steep for ¹/₂ hour, strain, and take 1–2 ounces per day.

Yarrow flowers help to stimulate the eliminative processes. Use 1 teaspoon to 1 cup boiling water and steep for 5–10 minutes. Drink 4 cups per day.

Horseradish, freshly ground or eaten raw, will help the body to eliminate excess fluids. Eat ¹/₂ cupful daily.

FALLING SICKNESS

Falling sickness is a form of epilepsy. Parsley, fennel, anise, and caraway will help to stimulate the body and prevent falling sickness. Use the roots, seeds, and leaves of any of these herbs, one herb at a time, mixing 1 ounce herb to 1 pint boiling water. Steep 5–10 minutes, strain, and take 4 ounces liquid morning and evening. After taking the tea, do not eat or drink anything for at least 3 hours. In addition, see the Brain section for more information.

GRAVES' DISEASE (PARKINSON'S DISEASE)
Make a tea using 2 ounces speedwell to 1 pint boiling water. Steep for 5–10 minutes and take 1 ounce daily.

MENINGITIS
Meningitis is an illness of the fluid that surrounds and protects the brain. It can be treated by shaving the back of the head and immersing the back of the head in a bowl of Epsom salts and warm water. This helps to draw out the inflammation. In addition, the patient should be given comfrey tea to drink. Make the tea using 1 teaspoon comfrey leaves to 1 cup boiling water. Steep 3–5 minutes, strain, and drink freely. Use at least 5 cups of the tea per day to help strengthen the system and fight the infection.

MULTIPLE SCLEROSIS AND MUSCULAR DYSTROPHY
Multiple sclerosis attacks the body in much the same way as muscular dystrophy does. It usually begins from the same basic reasons. Muscular dystrophy must be treated with raw fruits and vegetables and lots of vitamin F. Apple pits contain large quantities of vitamin F, and alfalfa supplies vitamin F as well as A, B, C, K, P, and G, and many minerals.

Each day for 1 week take only fresh fruit juices, some raw goat milk, and 1 slice sourdough bread. Drink only one type of juice each day. During the second week, eat only raw fruit for one meal and raw vegetables for the next, then raw fruit again, etc. Eat many different kinds of fruits and vegetables to ensure a proper supply of vitamins and minerals. Be sure to take only one type of fruit or fruit juice per day. Carrot, spinach, parsley, and cucumber juices are helpful. Continue with 1 slice sourdough bread per day.

Fast for 5 days, alternating fruit juice one day and vegetable juices the next. Thereafter, stay with a strict diet of raw fruit and vegetables for the next 2 weeks. Place an emphasis on keeping the system alkaline. After the first 5 days, add to the diet some sprouted wheat and 1 slice per day sourdough bread. This diet will help to rebuild the nervous system and stimulate the metabolism. Smoking and drinking alcoholic beverages must be eliminated entirely. Also eliminate coffee, any form of sugar, and all white flour or bread products except the prescribed sourdough bread.

To make a tonic for degenerative diseases, cut up 1 pound unpeeled raw beets and cover with $1/4$ pound each brown sugar and natural honey. Allow mixture to stand for 48 hours. Take 1 ounce morning and evening every day until condition is completely cleared.

American century is a good herb to take while recovering from degenerative diseases because it helps to build up the body. Use 1 teaspoon herb to 1 cup boiling water and steep for $1/2$ hour. Drink 2 cups of the cold tea per day.

PALSY
To treat palsy, use the raw beet tonic just given.

Sage tea helps to quiet the tremors of the limbs. Use 1 teaspoon herb to 1 cup boiling water and steep for 5–10 minutes. Sip slowly 3–5 cups per day or as needed.

Five to six grains of black cohosh, taken daily, will help to control involuntary spasms of palsy and St. Vitus' dance.

Chickweed leaf ointment will help to stop the tremor of the limbs. Apply to the legs to treat varicose veins. Use 1 ounce leaves combined with 1 pound cocoa butter or paraffin. Warm until mixed and then allow to steep for several minutes. Apply to affected parts after it is cool enough.

Fit root is a good treatment for fainting and spasms of all kinds. Use 1 teaspoon fit root and 1 teaspoon fennel seed in 1 pint boiling water. Steep for 20 minutes and drink 1–2 cups per day.

PARALYSIS

Paralysis is caused by a block in the flow of blood to a particular organ or limb. Care should be taken to ensure that the system is kept clean and functioning properly. Here are some herbs that help in the treatment of paralysis.

Paralysis of the tongue may be treated with ginger leaf tea. Use one or two leaves or 1 teaspoon dried leaves to 1 cup boiling water. Drink hot. Sip 2 cups per day.

Prickly ash is a good treatment for paralysis of the tongue and mouth. Use 1 ounce bark or leaves to 1 pint boiling water, steep for 15 minutes, and drink 3–4 cups per day.

Snake root will stimulate the system and help to remove blockages. Use $1/2$–1 teaspoon root to 1 cup boiling water, steep 3 minutes, and sweeten with honey. Take 1–3 cups per day.

Lecithin, which is contained in every cell in the brain and spinal column, can help to dissolve blockages that cause paralysis. Take 1 tablespoon in liquid, powder, granules, or capsule form daily.

POLIO

To treat polio, take 600 mg. each of vitamins C and P (hesperidin) per day until the capillary activity is improved. Vitamin P is found in the white part of the skin of all citrus fruits. Eat plenty of bioflavonoids, which are found in berries, currents, plums, apricots, and lemons.

Green peppers are a rich source of vitamins and minerals and are very good for helping to treat polio.

Coughs and Colds

Coughs, colds, and sore throats, all indicate congestion in the system. Do not eat or drink any milk or milk products because they are acid and mucous forming. Goat or soy milk products may be substituted; these products are alkaline and nonmucous forming. To treat these conditions, you must clear the congestion in the body, and a juice or other liquid diet for several days will help to clean the digestive tract and relieve the cold. Drinking a quart of fruit juice a day is a good way to build up body resistance and to prevent colds. Here are other ways of relieving these conditions.

ALLERGIES AND HAY FEVER

Allergic reactions are caused when the antigen production of the liver, pancreas, and spleen exceed the normal production. This condition indicates a lack of vitamin C, calcium, and magnesium. Sugars, and all sugar products, further deplete these nutrients, and milk and milk products clog the system. Allergies and hay fever conditions can be controlled by eliminating all nonnutritious foods from the diet and by building the body resistance to a level that can strengthen the system. Canned foods should be replaced with a diet of fresh fruits and vegetables and especially fruits with pits in them. Eat plenty of foods rich in vitamin C, such as apricots, peaches, and cherries.

Red clover helps to build up the body resistance to allergies. Use 1 teaspoon blossoms to 1 cup boiling water and steep for 5–10 minutes. Drink 3–4 cups per day before coming in contact with allergy or hay fever causes. During the season, or if an attack occurs, double your intake of tea, and take large amounts of vitamin C per hour. Rosehips supply the most easily assimilated sources of vitamin C.

Farum phos, a cell salt, is good for treating hay fever. Dissolve three small tablets on the tongue every 2 hours for the first day, and thereafter three times a day.

Licorice helps to build up resistance to allergens. Use 3 roots of licorice to 1 quart water. Boil together for 10 minutes, strain, and take 1 tablespoon three times per day every other day for a 6-day period.

ASTHMA, BRONCHITIS, AND CHEST INFECTIONS
Blue violet leaf tea will help to dry out the moisture in the

lungs that activates asthma attacks. Use 1 teaspoon leaves to 1 cup boiling water and drink 2 cups daily. Continue for several months to help completely dry the lungs.

Masterwort helps to control asthma by stimulating the activity of the lungs. Use 1 ounce masterwort to 1 pint boiling water and steep for 10 minutes. Take $^{1}/_{2}$ cup three times a day.

Honeysuckle is a good treatment for asthmatic conditions. Use $^{1}/_{2}$ teaspoon honeysuckle to 1 cup boiling water and take 1 cup three to four times a day.

Jerusalem artichokes contain vitamins A, B_1, B_2, and C and will nourish the lungs and helped to relieve asthmatic conditions. Eat raw or in soups or salads.

Prickly ash helps to remove obstructions from the system and will help to clear the lungs. Use $^{1}/_{2}$ teaspoon prickly ash to 1 pint boiling water. Drink 4 or more cups per day.

Apricots contain many nutrients that promote healing of lung conditions such as tuberculosis (TB), bronchitis, and asthma. Eat 3–6 apricots daily.

Vitamin E promotes healing of the lungs and helps to rebuild cells. Asthmatic sufferers should eat foods that are high in vitamin E and take supplements daily. Start with a low dosage and, over a period of several weeks, increase up to 1,200 IU per day.

Pennyroyal will help asthmatic congestion. Use 1 teaspoon

leaves and flowers in 1 cup boiling water. Sweeten with honey to taste and take 1 teaspoon twice a day.

Yerba mate will help to control pain in the lungs and increase respiratory capacity. Use $1/2$ teaspoon yerba mate to 1 cup boiling water, and take 3–5 cups per day.

Cockleburr tea is a good treatment for asthma. Steep 2 handfuls in 1 quart boiling water and drink 1 cup four times a day.

Two handfuls of wild plum bark steeped in a quart of boiling water helps to control asthma attacks. Take 1–2 cups daily.

To help sleep, asthmatics may sleep on a pillow stuffed with life everlasting herb.

Speedwell helps to eliminate obstructions in all parts of the body, including the lungs. Use 2 ounces to 1 pint boiling water, and take $1/2$ ounce per day.

For asthma, mix equal parts garlic, ginseng, magnesium, and vitamin C. Take $1/2$ teaspoon of the combined mixture before each meal. This remedy is not recommended for women because of the use of ginseng.

Boil three licorice roots in 1 pint water and sip throughout the day for asthma.

To treat bronchial asthma, mix onions, honey, and skunk cabbage or garlic. Steep mixture with enough water to make a tea and drink 1 cup daily.

Bronchial asthma sufferers should abstain from all meat, eggs, bread, and milk products; these products will create more mucous in the system.

Mix 2 tablespoons ground flax seeds with 1 pint boiling water, simmer for 2 or 3 minutes, strain, and sip slowly. This tea helps clear out mucous from bronchial tubes and colds.

Vervain promotes perspiration, which helps the body to expel phlegm and bronchial mucous. Use 1 teaspoon herb and 1 cup boiling water to make a tea. Steep 3–5 minutes, strain, and sip 1–2 cups per day. This herb works quickly.

White bryony helps to cleanse mucous from the lungs. It is useful for treating pneumonia, tonsilitis, glandular swelling, and all bronchial ailments. Use 1 ounce powdered bryony to 1 pint boiling water and take 1 tablespoon morning and evening. Continue daily for up to 6 months, or as long as needed. Asthma and emphysema patients should not exceed the recommended dosage; the condition must be treated slowly to allow time for the lungs to replace diseased cells.

For bronchitis, mix $1/2$ ounce each of hyssop, comfrey, and coltsfoot with 1 pint boiling water and steep for 10 minutes. Drink $1/2$ cup twice a day. For severe conditions, take up to 3 cups a day.

For flu and bronchial ailments, use 1 teaspoon blue violet leaves to 1 cup boiling water. Steep for 2–3 minutes and sip slowly. Drink 2–3 cups daily to help remove mucous.

Fenugreek will help to expel phlegm and cleanse the kidneys. Use 1 teaspoon to 1 pint boiling water and drink ¹/₂ cup tea twice a day. Continue for several weeks until mucous is gone.

Vitamin A is helpful in all bronchial troubles. Fresh parsley, watercress, and alfalfa are good sources of this vitamin.

Dry nettle leaves help to purify the blood and dissolve mucous in the lungs and glands. It is also used to cleanse the stomach of undigested food. Use 1 teaspoon leaves to 1 cup boiling water and drink ¹/₂ cup three times a day.

Mayflower herb is a good decongestant and will help to control mucous in the nasal cavity. Use 1 teaspoon herb to 1 cup boiling water and drink ¹/₂ cup three times a day.

To treat flu, colds, chest infections, and malaria, bake a lemon in the oven until it splits open. Beat the lemon juice with 1 tablespoon grape brandy and 2 pinches of salt. After taking a hot bath, before retiring drink the mixture and take 10 drops jaborandi in a cup of hot water. After 6 hours, sponge down and rub the body with oil.

Mullein flower tea is a good treatment for chest and bronchial ailments. Use 1 teaspoon flowers to 1 pint boiling water. Take 1 tablespoon three times a day to loosen phlegm.

Cooked barley mixed with lemon and water is a good treatment for bronchitis. Liquify the mixture in a blender and sip slowly.

To expel mucous, mix the juice of 1 Spanish onion, 1 teaspoon salt, and $1/2$ glass water and gargle.

Dandelion is an effective blood cleanser and body purifier. It contains plenty of vitamin C, which promotes healing of tuberculosis. Use 1 teaspoon herb to 1 cup boiling water and drink at least 3 cups per day.

Garlic is the most common blood purifier. One bulb per day will build resistance to tuberculosis and help to clear up the condition once contracted.

Apricots help to supply nutrients needed by TB patients. Eat 3–5 daily.

Horehound leaves are a good mucous expectorant. When this herb is boiled down to syrup form, it may be used to treat colds, coughs, asthma, and TB. The tea may be used to promote perspiration and urination. Use 1 teaspoon leaves to 1 cup boiling water and steep for 5 minutes. Sip slowly over a period of several hours.

To Avoid Contagious Disease
Hold juniper berries under the tongue to protect yourself from contagious diseases. They may be changed when soggy. The berries help to prevent infection from entering the body. Make dittany into a tea and rub onto the body to help protect against contagion.

Alfalfa tea, taken daily, will help to build up the body resistance to disease. The tablets may be used instead of the tea.

EMPHYSEMA

Emphysema is a bronchial condition that is characterized by excess mucous in the lungs. White bryony is good for clearing this congestion. Use 1 ounce bryony powder to 1 pint boiling water and take 1 tablespoon twice a day. In severe cases, the dosage may be increased to three times a day. Do not exceed this dosage because the lungs must be cleared gradually in order to replace damaged cells. Use only white bryony and continue treatment for 6 months or more until condition is completely cleared.

Blue violet leaves are also good for emphysema. Use 1 teaspoon to 1 cup boiling water and steep for 2–3 minutes. Drink 2–3 cups per day.

FEVER

*To reduce fever, squeeze the juice from one grapefruit and put aside in the refrigerator. Cut up the grapefruit pulp and boil for 10 minutes in 8 ounces of distilled water. Strain and combine with the juice from the refrigerator. Sip slowly to bring down fever. For intermittent fevers or flu use six grapefruits and 48 ounces distilled water. Sip slowly throughout the day. Do not eat or drink anything else except water. Continue for 2–3 days or as long as necessary.

To treat fever of influenza, use 2 teaspoons peach tree leaves in 1 cup boiling water. Cool, strain, and take 1 tablespoon every hour.

Combine 1 ounce feverweed and 1 pint boiling water to make a tea. Drink freely instead of water to bring down fever.

The fresh bark of button bush is good for recurring fever. Make a tea using ½ teaspoon root or bark and 1 cup boiling water. Add 1 teaspoon honey and boil until the mixture is syrupy. Take 1 teaspoon every hour.

For fever and fatigue, combine 5–20 grains cayenne with 1 quart boiling water for 10 minutes. Add 1 teaspoon honey and 1 cup orange juice. This treatment will help reduce fever and restore equilibrium. Sip slowly.

MONONUCLEOSIS

Mono, or the kissing disease, is caused by a combination of nervous and physical exhaustion due to a lack of proper nutrients in the diet and an excess of stress. In the early stages, it may be contagious, hence its secondary name.

For mono, take 1 clove chopped garlic in 1 teaspoon olive oil first thing in the morning. Eat no food until the bowels move, and repeat the next day. Take only vegetable juices for the next 2 days, particularly carrot, celery, spinach, or parsley juice. Take apple or pumpkin juice for days 3 and 4. Drink about 8 ounces of liquid each hour during these 4 days, and repeat this diet until condition is cleared. This stimulates the entire system to eliminate blockages caused by devitalized foods.

PNEUMONIA

Warm ½ cup goose grease and have the patient drink it. Give lemon to help get rid of the taste. Place a hot water bottle at the feet and cover the patient well. During the night, the patient will sweat heavily. Witnesses of this treatment say that the pneumonia will be gone in the morning.

Giant Solomon's seal is a good treatment for chest infections. Take in a tea and make into a poultice. Use only the root. For tea use 1 teaspoon to 1 cup boiling water and drink 3 cups per day. Change the poultice when dry and reapply.

To control bleeding of the lungs, mix 2 ounces slippery elm bark with 1 quart warm milk. Take 1 teaspoon every $1/2$ hour to soothe the membranes of the lungs.

Rub oil of cloves into the chest to treat all chest ailments. This will help to break tension and clear breathing passages. Give 1 drop oil of cloves with 1 teaspoon honey once or twice a day. This treatment is also effective for tuberculosis.

SORE THROATS

For sore throats, slowly roast a ripe lemon in the oven until it cracks open, and take 1 teaspoon of the juice with a little honey once every hour. This mixture is also good for hacking coughs.

To reduce swelling from sore throats, make a poultice using cudweed and cover with plastic. Change the poultice 2–3 times a day.

Make a tea using $1/2$ teaspoon mouseroot in 1 cup boiling water to use as a gargle for mouth irritations. Gargle twice a day and drink the remaining tea.

Queen's delight and sundew herbs help to control coughing and laryngitis. Use 1 teaspoon herbs to 1 cup boiling water, and drink 1 cup twice a day.

Mix 4 tablespoons cider vinegar and 1 pint boiling water to make a good, antiseptic mouthwash. Gargle several times a day.

Sage tea is an excellent gargle for sore throats. Use morning and evening and when needed throughout the day. Use 1 teaspoon sage to 1 cup boiling water, steep several minutes, and strain. Drink remainder of the tea.

*Gargle with diluted lemon juice 1 hour and black tea the next hour alternately all day to help clear sore throats and laryngitis. Do not drink the black nonherbal tea, but the tannic acid it contains is good for soothing the throat when used intermittently with the lemon and warm water.

Arsesmart helps to clear up thrush (mouth ulcers) and is a soothing gargle for sore throats. Use 1 ounce leaves to 1 pint cold water. Drink 3 ounces when thirsty in place of water. As a gargle, use 3–5 times per day.

Garlic is a good treatment for colds and hacking coughs. Eat one bulb daily.

Balm tea helps to soothe the throat and strengthen the voice for singing. Use 1 teaspoon leaves to 1 cup boiling water, steep 3–5 minutes, and add 1 teaspoon honey. Sip slowly, repeating as needed.

Cooked barley mixed with lemon and water helps to soothe sore throats. Use enough water to liquify the mixture and gargle when needed.

Bush honeysuckle made into a tea is a good gargle for sore throats. Use $^1/_4$ teaspoon to 1 cup boiling water. Gargle several times a day.

Mix equal parts yarrow, elderberry, and peppermint and make into a tea using 1 teaspoon combined herbs to 1 cup boiling water. This tea helps cleanse the system of congestion and stimulates elimination; take freely at the first sign of a cold.

Pennyroyal tea is good for coughs and colds. Make the tea using 1 teaspoon leaves to 1 cup boiling water and drink several cups per day.

Avens herb is a good treatment for fever, colds, and sore throats. Make a tea using 1 teaspoon to 1 pint boiling water. Drink 3 cups per day.

Clover tonic is good for all bronchial ailments and colds, and it helps to build up the body's resistance to disease. Steep 1 teaspoon clover in 1 cup boiling water and drink often during the day.

Bayberry tea helps cleanse the throat of putrid substances. Use 1 teaspoon bayberry to 1 cup boiling water and steep for 30 minutes. Gargle often until the condition improves. Drink a pint of the lukewarm tea to thoroughly cleanse the stomach and help to restore normal mucous production.

Thyme tea helps to prevent colds and infections. Use 1 teaspoon herb to 1 cup boiling water and drink freely throughout the day.

Comfrey tea, prepared using 1 teaspoon leaves to 1 cup boiling water, helps promote healing of colds and infection. Drink 4 or more cups per day.

Make a tea using 1 teaspoon St. John's wort to 1 cup boiling water. Drink and go to bed. The herb will induce perspiration and help to control coughing.

Angelica root is an expectorant and will help to control coughs, colds, and all bronchial ailments. Use $^1/_4$ teaspoon root to 1 pint boiling water. Drink slowly, several cups per day.

Eat small amounts of grated horseradish mixed with honey to help control hoarseness.

For swollen throat glands, use a poultice of crushed ground ivy leaves. Cover the poultice with a piece of plastic to keep the heat in and change when dry.

A tea using 1 teaspoon bull rushes root to 1 cup boiling water helps control chronic coughs. Drink $^1/_2$ cup three times a day.

Parsnips are a good treatment for shortness of breath and coughs. Use 1 teaspoon root to 1 cup boiling water and drink 2 cups per day.

Lungwort is a good treatment for coughs and to expel

mucous. Boil 1 ounce dried leaves and 1 pint milk in a double boiler for 10 minutes. Other cooking processes will cause constipation. Sweeten with honey to taste and sip often to ease throat congestion.

American cowslip tea is a mucous expectorant that is useful for colds and chronic chest congestion. Use 1 teaspoon cowslip to 1 cup boiling water to make a tea. Steep 5–10 minutes and drink 2 cups per day.

Use the entire wild evening primrose plant to make a tea to treat coughs and colds. Use 1 teaspoon herb, cut into small pieces, in 1 cup boiling water. Drink the cold tea slowly throughout the day.

Ginger leaf tea will help to stop colds at the onset. Use 1 teaspoon ginger to 1 cup boiling water and drink hot, $1/2$ cup at a time. Ginger warms the body and stimulates circulation.

Dandelion tea helps to clear cold infections. Use 1 teaspoon greens to 1 cup boiling water and drink freely.

Monkshood is a good treatment for fevers, colds, and coughs, and to ease bronchial congestion. The powdered root, mixed with egg white and applied to the chest, helps to draw out the congestion. Remove when dry and repeat if necessary.

Dill tea, used 1 teaspoon herb to 1 cup boiling water, is good for coughs. Drink 2 cups per day.

To help relieve colds and sniffles, press the juice of grated black horseradish and mix with up to $^1/_2$ pound honey. Take 2 tablespoons before each meal and 1 hour before bedtime.

Chervil is a good treatment for coughs. Make a tea using 1 teaspoon herb to 1 cup boiling water. Take 1 tablespoon three times a day.

Coltsfoot is a helpful remedy for colds and coughs. Use 1 teaspoon leaves to 1 cup boiling water and steep for $^1/_2$ hour. Drink freely.

Cayenne is recommended for people who have been exposed to colds and as a treatment for already established colds. Take 5–20 grains in warm water or in capsule form. Do not exceed recommended dosage; excess cayenne can irritate the mucous membranes of the digestive tract.

Bloodroot is a mucous expectorant and is a good treatment for colds. Use $^1/_{12}$ grain to 1 pint water. Take 1 teaspoon three times a day.

Pleurisy root is a good treatment for colds, flu, fever, asthma, and chest infections of all kinds. Use 1 teaspoon powdered root in 1 cup boiling water. Drink 4–5 cups per day.

SINUSITIS
Blueberries, carrots, and cucumbers are all good for stuffy sinuses. They may be eaten fresh or juiced.

Fresh ground ivy tea will help to relieve nasal congestion and stop headaches. Use 1 teaspoon leaves to 1 cup boiling water.

When cooled, sniff up the nose.

Take two tablets of garlic and parsley every 4 waking hours for 6 days. This helps to clear up chronic sinus trouble.

Mix chopped onions and garlic and eat to help soothe the mucous lining of the nose and sinuses. This treatment also kills any harmful bacteria in the nose and mouth.

Garlic helps to control nicotine poisoning and helps in the treatment of all respiratory infections including sinusitis. Take 1 bulb per day.

Pour a strong tea of melilot herb over the head after washing the hair to help clear up sinus conditions.

To help soothe and clean the sinuses, follow this diet for 4 days. Thereafter, eat horseradish once a week with fish and rice. Be sure to take at least three 8-ounce glasses of water per day and abstain from all milk and milk products.

On day 1, drink 6 ounces spinach juice and 10 ounces carrot juice.

On day 2, eat 1 pint horseradish with one whole lemon.

On day 3, drink 10 ounces carrot juice and 3 ounces each beet and cucumber juice.

On day 4, drink 1 pint carrot juice.

For all sinus conditions, massage underneath the big toe on both feet and each of the toes as well. Repeat daily.

Take a spoonful of honey with 2 drops eucalyptus oil to help clear sinuses. Take just before retiring.

Vitamin A promotes healthy functioning of the nasal cavity, sinuses, and the entire respiratory tract. A lack of vitamin A can lower resistance to infections in these areas. Eat plenty of chickweed, alfalfa, and parsley to supply these nutrients.

Make an ointment using chickweed or archangel and lanolin. Use the herb in powder form. Apply the ointment to the face, let dry, and repeat. This treatment helps shrunken sinuses become more pliable.

To clear the sinuses, take a warm bath and abstain from all milk products. Mix grated horseradish with lemon juice to make a thick sauce. Take 1 teaspoon mixture morning and evening to help clear nasal congestion. Do not eat or drink anything for 1 hour before or after taking the mixture.

Horehound leaves are a good mucous expectorant. Use 1 tea-spoon to 1 cup boiling water, steep, and sip over a period of several hours. In addition, the syrup made from boiling the leaves and roots helps to treat colds, coughs, asthma, sinusitis, and tuberculosis. Take 1 teaspoon syrup daily until the condition is cleared.

Digestive System

Each organ of the digestive system — the mouth, throat, stomach, and intestines — is dependent upon the preceding organ to have done its job properly. A malfunction in one organ will drastically affect the functioning of the others.

AIDS TO DIGESTION

The body manufactures certain enzymes that break down starches and modify proteins to prepare them for use by the body. Some of these enzymes are found in brewer's yeast, raw honey, pollen, rosehips, and kelp. Papayas are particularly high in protein-modifying enzymes. Eating adequate amounts of these foods will boost production of digestive enzymes.

Plaintain soothes and tones the internal organs. Use 1 teaspoon to 1 cup boiling water, and drink 2 cups per day for 3–4 days.

Mix bileberry with equal parts thyme, strawberry leaves, and hyssop. Use 1 teaspoon herbs mixed with 1 cup boiling water and drink cold. This tea soothes the bowels and helps increase the body's resistance to disease.

Agrimony is good for all digestive disorders. Use in capsule or powder form and take 5 grains three times a day.

Burdock is good for all digestive disorders. Use 1 teaspoon herb to 1 cup boiling water and steep for 10 minutes. Drink 3 cups per day.

Cinnamon helps tone the bowels. Use $1/4$ teaspoon cinnamon in 1 cup boiling water. Take 1 cup per day.

THE MOUTH

The mouth is the first organ of the digestive system. If you chew properly, the food you swallow will already be partially digested and the body will already have begun to assimilate the vitamins and minerals contained in the food.

For water brash (burping foods or liquids into the mouth), chew a small piece of calamus slowly and swallow the juice to help bring relief. Children should be given a weak tea made with ¹/₂ teaspoon calamus to 1 cup boiling water. Give only cooled tea to children.

Arsesmart herb is an excellent gargle for thrush (mouth ulcers) and sore throats. Use 1 ounce leaves in 1 pint cold water. Drink 3 ounces when thirsty in place of water, or gargle 3–5 times per day. This tea is an antibiotic that has no side effects.

Charcoal sweetens the breath and aids the digestive system by absorbing odors and gas.

For halitosis, mix 1 teaspoon aromatized sodium perborate with ¹/₂ glass warm water. Rinse out the mouth in the morning and evening. Do not swallow.

Chlorophyl, found in all green plants, helps absorb breath odors. Eat fresh parsley, watercress, or chickweed when needed.

THE THROAT
Sage tea is an excellent gargle for sore throats. Use 1 teaspoon sage to 1 cup boiling water. Steep for several minutes and strain. Gargle and sip morning and evening as needed.

Gargle with pure (or diluted) lemon juice, and then gargle with black tea an hour later. Keep alternating throughout the day to relieve sore throat and laryngitis. Do not drink the black nonherbal tea, but the tannic acid it contains is good for soothing the throat when used as directed with the lemon.

THE STOMACH

Bloodroot helps to stimulate the gastric and intestinal secretions and aids digestion. Use $1/12$ grain to 1 cup boiling water and sip slowly. Take 2 cups per day.

Buckbean root is good for improving digestion. Make a tea using 1 teaspoon root to 1 cup boiling water. Slowly swallow a large mouthful three times a day. This tea is bitter but effective.

Use 1 ounce prickly ash in 1 pint boiling water to make a stomach tonic. Steep the mixture 15 minutes and drink 3–4 cups per day.

Lovage is useful for all disorders of the stomach and urinary tract. Use 1 teaspoon herb to 1 cup boiling water and drink 4 cups per day.

Ground ivy is a good treatment for lead colic. Use 1 teaspoon ivy to 1 cup boiling water and drink 2 cups per day.

Garlic will help to relieve gas, heartburn, stomach upset, and all forms of indigestion; it destroys dangerous organisms in the system without harming the necessary bacteria.

Stomach Cramps

*Parsley tea will help to relieve stomach cramps. Make a tea using 1 teaspoon fresh or dried parsley to 1 cup boiling water. Steep 4–5 minutes and sip slowly.

To help soothe stomach cramps, make a tea using 1 teaspoon valarian root or leaves to 1 cup boiling water. Drink 2–3 cups per day.

St. John's wort helps stomach pain. Use $^1/_2$ teaspoon wort to 1 cup boiling water, and drink 1 cup three times a day.

Stomach Ulcers

Ulcers are usually caused by tension. If you will reorganize your life to eliminate heavy pressure and stress, many ulcers will disappear. Vitamins A, C, and E will soothe stomach ulcers. It is always more beneficial to get the vitamins you need from the food you eat rather than from supplements. See the appendices for lists of foods that are high in these vitamins.

Stomach disorders will respond to raw juices, particularly carrot, celery, cabbage, tomato, and parsley. Use few or no spices. Vitamin E should be added to the diet to help clear up all stomach conditions.

Cucumber juice is good for stomach and bladder ulcers. Drink several cups a day.

A strict diet of avocados will help to heal ulcers. For 2 weeks, eat nothing but avocados and sip at least 3 glasses of water per day.

Carrot juice is nourishing and soothing for stomach ulcers. Drink $1/2$ cup three times a day.

Parsley juice and alfalfa promote healing of ulcers. Drink 1 cup parsley juice morning and evening, or take 1 tablespoon parsley 3–4 times a day. Alfalfa tablets may be taken morning and evening after meals.

Papayas contain enzymes that replenish the stomach lining and help with protein digestion. Make a tea using $1/2$ teaspoon powder or root to 1 cup boiling water. Steep several minutes and drink 1 cup per day. This tea is particularly beneficial if you eat large quantities of meat.

Balm helps to relieve chronic stomach conditions, including ulcers. Make a tea using $1/2$ teaspoon to 1 pint boiling water. Steep several minutes, strain, and drink 3 cups per day.

Mix gentian, wormwood, comdurango, and American century in equal parts. Use 1 teaspoon mixture to 1 cup boiling water and steep for 3–5 minutes. Drink 2 cups per day for ulcers.

Green elder bark tea will promote healing of ulcers. Use 1 teaspoon bark to 1 cup boiling water and steep for 5 minutes. Strain and drink 3 cups per day.

Barley helps to rebuild the lining of the stomach and soothes stomach ulcers because it contains vitamins B_1 and B_2.

For ulcers, take $1/2$ teaspoon powdered cloves or $1/2$ teaspoon oil of cloves. Hold in the mouth until dissolved and mixed well with the saliva. Repeat this treatment three times per day.

Take 1 teaspoon concentrated licorice syrup daily and eat foods high in B_{12} (see appendices for sources). Continue treatment daily for ulcers.

Comfrey and pepsin are recommended for ulcerative colitis. They will help soothe the digestive tract and dissolve mucous from the walls of the intestines. Make a tea with 1 teaspoon mixed comfrey and pepsin to 1 cup boiling water and set aside. Boil 3 tablespoons flaxseed in 1 pint of water for 5 minutes and strain. Add the comfrey-pepsin tea and drink at once.

Persimmons are a high energy food and will promote healing of ulcers by soothing the mucous membranes in the digestive tract. Eat one persimmon a day.

The following diet is recommended for treatment of peptic ulcers:

On day 1, eat nothing and drink 1 pint fresh carrot juice.

On day 2, eat nothing, drink 10 ounces carrot juice, 3 ounces spinach juice, and 2 ounces parsley juice.

On day 3, eat nothing, drink 1 pint each spinach juice, celery juice, and carrot juice.

INTESTINES
COLIC
Colic is caused by gas in the system. The child may have gotten this from the mother, or, when formula is used, it indicates that the mixture is too rich for the child's system. Soy

milk formulas can cause colic also, if the mixture needs more dilution.

Horsebain herb helps to relieve colic. Use 1 teaspoon powdered leaves to 1 cup boiling water. Give $^1/_2$–1 cup cooled mixture when needed.

*Camomile tea is a good treatment for colic. Use $^1/_4$ teaspoon flowers to 1 cup boiling water and steep for 5–10 minutes. Sweeten with honey and give warm. Test for temperature.

Lovage tea helps ease the pain of colic. Use $^1/_4$ teaspoon herb to 1 cup boiling water and steep for 3 minutes. Give $^1/_2$ cup cooled mixture. Sweeten with honey if desired.

CONSTIPATION

Proper elimination is absolutely necessary for good health. When nutritive supplies are insufficient, the body lacks the energy needed to evacuate the bowels as completely and frequently as necessary. If your body is in good condition and you are eating the proper foods, you should have three bowel movements per day. Foods that are high in vitamins A, B, C, E, G, and K will help to relieve constipation. These vitamins are found in large quantities in cashews, Jerusalem artichokes, spinach, prunes, persimmons, mangoes, bell peppers, cranberries and cranberry juice, cucumbers, asparagus, green beans, bamboo shoots, and all roughage foods such as bean sprouts and lettuce.

A pantothenic acid deficiency can cause constipation and

other digestive disorders. Pantothenic acid is found in royal jelly, honey, human milk, peanuts, broccoli, and most other vegetables.

DIARRHEA

Diarrhea is a symptom and not a disease. It indicates that the body is ridding itself of intruding organisms or excessive wastes from overeating.

Garlic will destroy harmful bacteria, but will not destroy beneficial bacteria found in the intestinal tract. Use in tea or eat raw in salads.

Cold raspberry leaf tea is an excellent treatment for diarrhea. Use 1 ounce leaves to $^1/_2$ pint water, simmer together for 20 minutes. Drink cold. Use $^1/_2$ ounce herb to $^1/_2$ pint water to treat diarrhea in babies.

Use 1 teaspoon ginger root to 1 cup boiling water, and take 3 cups per day for diarrhea.

Apricots help to check diarrhea. Eat three whole apricots per day.

Swamp dogwood is a good treatment for diarrhea and dyspepsia. Make into a tea using 1 teaspoon leaves or bark in 1 cup boiling water. Drink 3 cups per day.

Use 1 ounce powdered slippery elm in 1 quart boiling water and simmer down to 1 pint. Take 1 teaspoon every $^1/_2$ hour to soothe the membranes of the intestinal tract. Honey may be added if needed. For infants or elderly people, cover powdered slippery elm with milk and eat like cereal.

Peruvian rhatany is a useful treatment for diarrhea to restore normal functioning of the bowels. Use $1/2$ teaspoon powdered root to 1 cup boiling water and take 2 cups per day.

Blueberries and huckleberries will help to relieve discomfort of diarrhea. Eat 5–20 fresh berries or bake in a pie made with honey.

Mix equal parts bileberry leaves, thyme, and strawberry leaves with 1 cup boiling water and drink cold to help control diarrhea. Honey may be added if necessary.

Make a tea using 1 teaspoon black elder bark or leaves and 1 cup boiling water. Sweeten with honey and take 1 cup per day to help diarrhea.

Barley is a body builder and will help to control diarrhea because it contains vitamins B_1 and B_2. Use in cereals, soups, and stews.

DYSENTERY

Dysentery can be treated with 2 tablespoons Epsom salts and 1 glass water. Drink quickly.

Boil whole Canada thistles in milk to make a soothing remedy for dysentery.

Juniper berries are helpful in the treatment of dysentery. Use five berries to 1 cup boiling water and drink $^1/_2$ cup twice a day.

GAS AND HEARTBURN

Gas is created when the food is not properly chewed and by drinking with meals; this process lessens the effectiveness of the salivary glands and impedes digestion. Eat slowly without liquids and relax while dining.

Gas may also be created by improper cooking. Beans contain many toxins that create gas if not properly cooked. To reduce the toxins and add to your enjoyment, here is a recipe for cooking beans:

> *Soak dried beans overnight and in the morning pour off the water. Add fresh water and 1 onion and bring to a boil. Strain off the water and throw out the onion. This wash will absorb the toxins in the beans that create gas. Replenish the water and add spices and herbs to taste. Cook until the beans are soft and well done. Eat only in small quantities; the body does not need excessive amounts of protein.*

Ginger, taken after a heavy meal, is an aid to digestion and helps prevent flatulence. Use $^1/_4$ teaspoon ginger to 1 cup hot water, steep 5 minutes, and sip slowly.

Angelica is a valuable treatment for digestive trouble. Use the following recipe. Grind into a powder and mix with 8 ounces pure alcohol. Let mixture stand for 8 days, then add 1 pound honey mixed with 2 $^1/_2$ pints tepid water. Take 1 tablespoon morning and evening to relieve gas.

>   *2 ounces angelica*
>   *¹/₄ ounce fennel*
>   *¹/₄ ounce anise*
>   *1 ounce coriander*

Catnip tea, taken warm, is helpful for gas. Use 1 pinch tea to ¹/₂ cup boiling water. Steep 5 minutes and then sip slowly when needed.

Fresh cleavers, when cooked with beans, adds flavor and minimizes production of gas.

Parsley is an efficient treatment for gas. Eat fresh and raw or make into a tea using 1 teaspoon to 1 cup boiling water.

Eat orange peels a few minutes after the meal to aid digestion.

Bay leaves make a pleasant tea that helps tone and strengthen the digestive organs and helps expel gas from both the stomach and the bowels. Use ¹/₂ teaspoon leaves to 1 cup boiling water. Sip slowly.

Slippery elm bark neutralizes stomach acid and helps to absorb gases. It contains enzymes that help digestion. Make a tea using 1 teaspoon bark or powder to 1 cup boiling water. Sip slowly.

Combine ¹/₂ teaspoon wild clover, 1 teaspoon lemon juice, and 1 cup boiling water. Take 1 tablespoon of the tea 3–5 times a day for gas.

For indigestion, mix ground horseradish with as much cream as it will absorb and eat slowly.

Camomile tea helps soothe intestinal disorders, gas, and cramps. Use 1 teaspoon herb to 1 cup boiling water and drink several cups per day.

*Peppermint tea aids the digestive processes when taken 1 hour after a meal. Make a tea using 1 teaspoon leaves to 1 cup boiling water and sip slowly.

Make a tea using $^1/_2$ teaspoon each cardamom seed and meadowsweet or horehound herb with 1 cup boiling water. Steep 3–5 minutes and sip slowly for heartburn.

Dill weed contains oils that relax the stomach. Use 1 teaspoon seeds in 1 cup water, boil for 15 minutes, strain, and drink slowly. This tea will help absorb gas and stop hiccups.

Combine 1 ounce gentian root, $^1/_2$ ounce colombo root, and $^1/_2$ ounce skullcap and cover with 2 pints cold water. Simmer slowly for 20 minutes and drink 1 hour before and 2 hours after meals. This is an effective, gentle treatment for elderly people suffering from indigestion.

Unground mustard seeds are an excellent treatment for gastritis. Take one seed the first day, two the second day, three the third day, adding one seed per day until twenty seeds are being taken. Then reduce the number by one seed each day until back down to one. Swallow the seeds with water first thing in the morning on an empty stomach.

Allspice helps relieve gas from the upper intestinal tract. Use ¹/₂ teaspoon allspice to 1 cup boiling water and drink 1 cup per day, or chew ¹/₄ teaspoon allspice and swallow.

Simple indigestion and heartburn can be relieved by sipping the juice of one-half fresh lemon in 1 cup tepid water with 1 teaspoon soda. Drink the mixture immediately.

HEMORRHOIDS AND PILES

Hemorrhoids may be caused by pressure on the rectum from unassimilated bulk foods; often this pressure increases during pregnancy. But overeating is the most common cause. When you have eaten too much food, the body is unable to digest it properly and the fecal matter will remain hard and lumpy and strain the muscles and veins of the anus.

To relieve pain of hemorrhoids, apply a poultice of cottage cheese to the anus. Change poultice three times per day until relief is obtained.

Juniper berries are useful for treatment of hemorrhoids. Put 4–5 berries in 1 pint boiling water and steep for ¹/₂ hour. Drink 4 cups per day.

Pilewort is a useful treatment for hemorrhoids and will help draw the tissues together. Use 1 ounce herb to 1 pint boiling water and take ¹/₂ cup twice a day.

Blue flag juice eases the pain of piles and hemorrhoids. Use 10–20 drops juice in ¹/₂ cup water or 1 ounce powder to 1 pint water. Drink ¹/₂ cup three times per day.

Steep black elder flowers in olive oil for 2 weeks and rub onto the skin outside the anus to relieve pain.

Mullein flowers will help relieve hemorrhoid pain. Use 1 ounce powdered leaves in 1 pint milk. Boil for 10 minutes, strain, and drink 3 cups per day.

A clove of garlic placed in the rectum helps reduce swelling of hemorrhoids.

*Use fresh comfrey leaves in a poultice to draw tissues of hemorrhoids back into place and help relieve the pain. If you do not have fresh comfrey, use the dried root or leaves. Make a strong tea by pouring boiling water over the herb. Use the softened roots and leaves in the poultice and drink the tea. This procedure will help to clear hemorrhoids completely.

Soak a piece of cotton with papaya juice and place against the rectum to draw out the irritation and stop the bleeding of piles and hemorrhoids.

Soften sicklewort leaves with boiling water and make into a poultice. Place the poultice against the rectum to help stop bleeding of piles.

LAXATIVES
Yerba mate stimulates peristalsis and nourishes the intestinal tract. It is a high source of vitamin C. Take 1 teaspoon yerba mate to 1 cup boiling water and drink several cups per day.

*Dandelion is useful for all types of constipation and will help strengthen the stomach. Use fresh in salads or make a tea using 1 teaspoon root to 1 cup boiling water. Steep for $^1/_2$ hour and drink 1–2 cups daily.

Cascara bark helps tone the bowels and aids elimination. Take 1 tablespoon before bedtime in tablet or capsule form. Do not exceed dosage.

Wormwood is an excellent, fast-acting laxative. Use $^1/_2$ teaspoon wormwood to 1 cup boiling water and sip slowly. Do not drink more than 1 cup in a 24-hour period.

Black root is good for constipation. Use 1–2 teaspoons per cup boiling water. Steep for 10 minutes. Black root helps remove obstructions of the digestive tract.

Pumpkin seeds are excellent for constipation. Chew 1 teaspoon seeds per day. Pumpkin seeds are high in male hormones and are not recommended for women.

American senna is an effective laxative. Use 1 teaspoon leaves or 5 pods to 1 cup boiling water, let steep $^1/_2$ hour, and drink $^1/_2$ cup morning and evening.

Masterwort stimulates the digestive organs and absorbs gases from the intestines. Use $^1/_2$ teaspoon masterwort to 1 cup boiling water. Drink 1 cup per day.

Black elder bark is a good laxative. Use 1 teaspoon bark to 1 cup boiling water. Take 1 cup per day.

American bearsfoot root stimulates the glands, relieves pain, and is an effective laxative. Use 1 teaspoon root to 1 cup boiling water and take at bedtime.

Soak fresh cucumbers in kelp water overnight and drink in the morning before breakfast. This mixture relieves congestion that causes nausea and is an excellent laxative.

A lack of B vitamins will cause constipation. Eat one yeast cake per day for several months to tone the bowels and relieve constipation. Comfrey tea, papaya, and chlorophyll tablets are also helpful.

The inner bark of the white ash tree is a useful treatment for constipation. Steep a heaping teaspoon in 1 cup boiling water for 30 minutes and drink $1/2$ glass in the morning and in the evening.

Use 1 teaspoon each buckhorn bark, Indian senna pods, and bladder wrack in 2 cups boiling water. Steep 10 minutes, strain, and take $1/2$ cup morning and evening for 2 days for constipation.

Eating 2–3 fresh tomatoes daily before breakfast helps to keep the bowels regular.

May apples will soothe the bowels and relieve constipation. Use 1 teaspoon leaves to 1 pint boiling water and take 1 teaspoon per day.

Bamboo shoots may be used for constipation and intestinal poisoning. Eat raw or cover with boiling water for 10 minutes to soften. Eat about ¹/₂ cup per day.

Soak 1 tablespoon whole flaxseed and 1 tablespoon wheat bran in 1 cup vegetable broth overnight. In the morning heat, blend well, and drink. Do not strain or chew. This mixture will help to restore normal peristalsis rhythm. Do not use during a fast.

To soothe the intestines and restore regularity to the bowels, eat only tree-ripened figs and salads with a dressing made of lemon and apple juice for 1 day each week. Figs help to reestablish the acid-alkaline balance in the system and ease colitis.

Vervain helps to remove obstructions of the colon. Use 1 teaspoon powdered plant to 1 cup boiling water and drink 1 cup every hour until results are obtained.

Persimmons will soothe the digestive tract and help relieve constipation, colitis, and sore throats.

In an emergency, olive oil will help relieve constipation. Sip small amounts (up to 1 cup) throughout the day until results are obtained. Lemon juice may be taken to cut the oily taste.

Ears and Eyes

EARS

The ears are vital sensory organs and need adequate supplies of vitamins A and C. These vitamins are beneficial for ear infections, pain, or deafness. High sources of A and C are carrots, carrot juice, parsley, and all citrus fruits. See the appendices for further food information.

DEAFNESS
Raw garlic and onion juice taken internally once a day can help to restore hearing. Use about 2 ounces combined mixture daily.

Summer savory is excellent for deafness. Use 1 ounce herb to 1 pint boiling water, steep several minutes, and strain. Drink 3 cups daily.

Mullein flowers steeped in olive oil for 2 weeks will make a good ointment for deafness. Use 1 drop in each ear once a week and massage the outside of the ear, both back and front, daily. Angelica juice dropped into the ear is helpful for deafness. Put 1 drop in each ear once a week.

EARACHES AND INFECTIONS
*Ear infections may be treated by boiling 1 clove of garlic in 1/2 cup water until soft but not mushy. Lay cooled clove on the outside of the ear, but do not push it down the ear canal! Cover with a piece of clean cotton and hold in place with cellophane tape. Leave poultice for several days (changing daily) until infection is drawn out.

Make a strong tea of mullein flowers using 1 teaspoon to 1/2 cup boiling water. Mix 1 tablespoon mixture with 1 tablespoon olive oil and let stand overnight. Use 1 drop of this liquid in each ear twice a week to help ease the ache.

Devil's walking stick seeds, when crushed, yield an oil that aids earache pain. Use 1 drop in affected ear once a week.

One pinch of dried yarrow leaves and 1 tablespoon boiling water mixed together and steeped for 5 minutes helps both earaches and infections. Use 1 drop in each ear once a week until condition clears.

One drop garlic oil in each ear helps clear ear infections. Use warm, not hot, oil and repeat once a week.

EAR DISCHARGE
Combine equal quantities of black currant leaves, honeysuckle, horehound, and giant hyssop. Use 1 teaspoon to 1 cup boiling water. Put 1 drop warm liquid in each ear. *Do not use hot.* Repeat once a week to help clear discharge.

EAR MITES
One drop warmed Campho-Phenique in each ear is a good treatment for ear mites. After 1 week use a small amount (3–5 drops) hydrogen peroxide in affected ear and allow to drain. The mites will come out with the liquid.

EAR NOISE
Ringing in the ears can be treated with summer savory. Use 1/2 teaspoon herb to 1/2 cup boiling water and steep for several minutes. Mix 1 teaspoon of this mixture with 1 teaspoon oil of roses. When cool, place 1 drop of mixture in each ear to help ease the ringing sensation. Repeat once a week until hearing clears.

Massage the neck behind and in front of each ear, then pull

gently as directed by the numbers and arrows in Diagram 4. Repeat daily.

Diagram 4
EAR MASSAGE

EAR WAX

To soften ear wax deposits, press firmly but gently behind the ear and in front of the ear, and then pull the ear lobe up and down (see Diagram 4). This procedure also stimulates ear circulation and should be repeated daily.

EYES

The eyes are sensory organs and, as such, they need plenty of vitamin C. Deficiencies in any of the vitamins or minerals will show up first in the eyes as little "bloodshot" lines corresponding to the area of the body that is malfunctioning. Iris diagnosis, although not included here, is becoming more widely practiced as a method of early detection and prevention of disease.

BAGS UNDER EYES

*Bags under eyes can be caused by water retention, stress, or most commonly, loss of sleep. Make a poultice using black nonherbal tea bags, moistened and laid over the eyes. This will help draw out the dark circles. Grated potato, apple, papaya leaves, cucumber, or alfalfa will also draw out circles and relax tension behind the eyes.

BLACK EYES

To reduce swelling and bruises of black eyes, use equal parts
lard and salt in a poultice and place over the eyes. This stimulates the circulation, which helps the body eliminate dead and
bruised cells.

BLOODSHOT EYES

Bloodshot eyes, except when caused by wind exposure, usually indicate a need for more vitamin B in the system. Eat
sprouted grains, sunflower seeds, and other foods high in B-
complex vitamins daily.

CATARACTS AND GLAUCOMA

Cataracts indicate a deficiency of B vitamins, especially B_2
(riboflavin). One heaping teaspoon daily of this vitamin is an
effective treatment. Glaucoma and cataracts also indicate the
need for vitamins A, C, E, and rutin and calcium. A healthy
diet, including foods that contain these vitamins, plus daily
supplements will help to alleviate this condition.

Celandine (greater) has been used in the treatment of cataracts for hundreds of years. Press the leaves, collect the liquid,
and drop into the eye twice a day. Operations can often be
avoided with this treatment.

*Place the yellow side of a piece of organic orange peel over
the eye and leave overnight. On the second night, use the
white side of a fresh piece of organic orange peel. If the peel
over the eye creates a great deal of heat, remove it and try
again the next night. Continue each night, alternating the side

of the peel, until condition is cleared. Use fresh peel each night, and use only organic oranges because commercial oranges have been sprayed with chemicals.

For treatment of glaucoma, take daily supplements of vitamins A, C, B, and E, and calcium and apply goldenseal tincture to the cornea three times per day in a solution of 2 drops in 1 ounce warm water. This treatment is also good for ulcers of the cornea.

Glaucoma sufferers should not drink coffee because caffeine is hard on the blood vessels of the eyes. Dandelion coffee, which is made from the dried root of dandelion, may be substituted.

Rosehips are an excellent treatment for glaucoma and cataracts. Make a tea using 1 teaspoon to 1 cup boiling water and drink at least 3 cups per day.

CHAPPED EYELIDS
For chapped eyelids gently rub the eyelids with witch hazel on a cotton ball. Repeat 2–3 times per day.

CLEANSING BABIES' EYES
Mix together dried poppy flowers and lavender flowers in equal quantities. Use $1/2$ teaspoon mixture to 1 cup boiling water, steep 5 minutes, and strain. When mixture is cool use to cleanse eyes morning and evening as needed.

CYSTS ON THE EYES
*The white inner lining of the orange skin contains vitamins

F and P, which help dissolve eye cysts. Take 6 tablespoons hourly for 1 day and make a tea using 1 teaspoon orange skin to 1 cup boiling water to use as eye drops. Put 1 drop tea in the affected eye once or twice per day. This substance also helps reduce swelling. Use only organic oranges and continue until condition clears.

Cysts on the eye can be treated with 1 drop of your own urine from the first elimination of the morning. Dab generously but carefully on the cyst.

Alfalfa is excellent for treating blurred vision and other conditions of the eyes. Dissolve 1 tablet in 1 cup boiling water and put 1 drop cooled liquid in each eye daily.

DIMMING OF SIGHT
Slit open white willow bark or crush the leaves and collect the liquid. One drop of the sap morning and evening in each eye will reduce redness of the eyes and improve dimming eyesight. This treatment is also helpful for removing film over the eyes. Repeat daily until condition clears.

Cover dragon flowers with distilled water and let stand overnight. Use 1 drop liquid in each eye morning and evening to improve eyesight.

One clary seed, dropped into the eye, will float around inside the eye and clean infection and help remove film. The seed will work itself out when the cleansing is completed. Repeat this procedure several times a day for severe infections. Follow this treatment with 3–4 drops of pure, fresh cream in the eye to ease the inflammation of the mucous membranes.

EYE INFECTIONS

Mix together 1 teaspoon canned evaporated milk and 1 drop spirit of camphor. Put 1 drop mixture in each eye morning and evening to help clear eye infections.

Two drops pure flaxseed oil in each eye morning and evening will help clear eye infections.

Conjunctivitis can be cleared by eating goat milk yogurt and using yogurt in a poultice on the eyes daily. It helps to destroy bacteria in the system that cause the infection.

Pinkeye can be cleared almost overnight by using grated apple in a poultice placed over the eyes. Leave on for 20 minutes. Repeat daily if needed.

For eye infections, use a tea made with dried quince seeds. Use $1/4$ teaspoon in $1/2$ cup boiling water. Steep until cool, then put 1 drop in each eye morning and evening for 1 week to clear up infection.

One clary seed, placed into the eye, will help to work out foreign objects in the eye. It will work around the eye to draw out the object. Follow with 3–4 drops of pure, fresh cream in the eye to ease the inflammation of the mucous membranes. The seeds, made into tea, will help strengthen the eyes and remove film from the eyes. Use 1 teaspoon seeds to 1 cup boiling water and allow tea to stand overnight before drinking.

Calcium helps to cleanse the eyes when the pigment layers are inflamed. Make a solution with 2 mg. calcium dissolved in $^1/_2$ cup warm water. Wash the eyes with this liquid morning and evening for 1 week. Use warm solution each time.

IMPROVING VISION

Mix the following ingredients in a blender and drink slowly before meals. Continue for 2 weeks to help improve vision.

> $^1/_4$ cup grapefruit juice
> $^1/_4$ cup apple juice
> $^1/_4$ cup orange juice
> 2 tablespoons wheat germ oil
> 1 tablespoon unfiltered honey
> 2 tablespoons apple cider vinegar

Pour 1 quart boiling water over 1 cup fresh parsley to make a tonic for the eyes. Steep for 15 minutes, strain, and drink 3 cups per day. Keep this tonic refrigerated.

Calcium and vitamin D are helpful for both near- and far-sightedness. See the appendices for foods that contain these vitamins, and use daily.

Three teaspoons of sunflower seeds per day contain high amounts of vitamins necessary to help vision.

Vitamin E helps clear foggy vision. Start taking small doses and build up slowly over several weeks to 400–800 IU daily.

To help strengthen the eyes, just before bedtime place a lighted candle even with the top of the head and sit 1 $^1/_2$ feet away. Sit erect, with feet together. Hold the eyelids open with index fingers and look at the candle without blinking for 5 minutes. Don't wipe away the tears; wiping may bruise the eyes. Repeat this procedure for 5 minutes every other night for 2 weeks. Stop for 2 weeks and then begin again. Continue until vision is strengthened.

To improve the eyes, place the index fingers at the outside corners of the eyes and do not press. Squeeze the eyes and relax several minutes. This helps to build the muscles of the eyes (see Diagram 5).

Diagram 5
STRENGTHENING
EYE MUSCLES

To improve the eyes, use maidenhair and green ginger, $^1/_2$ teaspoon each with $^1/_2$ cup boiling water. Put 1 drop in each eye morning and evening until the eye film has cleared.

Rosemary tea helps to strengthen sight. Use 1 teaspoon rosemary to 1 cup boiling water and put 1 drop in each eye morning and evening. Drink the rest of the cup of tea.

*Sage tea helps keep the eyes bright and also improves the memory. Use 1 teaspoon sage to 1 cup boiling water and drink freely throughout the day. One cup daily for 6 months helps to clear and cleanse the eyes.

Tea made with juniper berries helps to strengthen sight. Use several berries to 1 cup boiling water. Drink 3 cups per day.

Rutin strengthens the eyes by helping to decrease capillary tension. Take 1 tablet (about 400 mg.) four times during the day.

NIGHT BLINDNESS

Watercress contains many vitamins and minerals that help restore night vision. Eat daily in salads or make into a tea using fresh herb.

Carrots and carrot juice help restore night vision. Eat 2–3 carrots per day or drink 4 ounces carrot juice.

RED EYES

Grapevine juice, a tiny drop in each eye, will help reddened eyes. The juice will sting but will help to clear the eyes quickly.

SORE AND INFLAMED EYES

Violet leaves, in tea and a poultice, help bring down swelling and draw out soreness from the eyes. Use 1 teaspoon leaves to 1 cup boiling water. Steep for 5 minutes, strain, and use strained leaves in a poultice on the eyes for 15 minutes. Drink the liquid.

Use grated or scraped raw Irish potatoes in a poultice on the eyes. This helps to relieve swelling or soreness. Use the poultice nightly for 15 minutes. This procedure may be repeated in the morning if needed.

Adder's-tongue herb made into a tea with horsetail herb is good for sore eyes. Use $^1/_2$ teaspoon each herb in 1 cup boiling water. Steep for 5 minutes and strain. Sip slowly 2 cups per day.

For sore eyes make an eye wash with the following ingredients. Combine herbs with water and steep for 20 minutes. Cool and wash eyes with the mixture each morning and evening until soreness is gone.

> $^1/_2$ *teaspoon fit root*
> $^1/_2$ *teaspoon fennel seed*
> *1 pint boiling water*

Swollen eyes can be soothed by making a poultice of grated apple and laying it over the eyes for 15–20 minutes. This will help draw out the swelling and relieve the irritation. Fresh corn silk, papaya, or witch hazel poultices may be used instead of apple.

*Lemon juice is a cleansing eyewash, especially when you have been exposed to dust, long hours under harsh lights, or work with printing compounds. This is a good all-around eyewash that will clean and soothe the eyes and help restore normal functioning. Use 1 drop lemon juice (fresh only!) in 1 eyecup (or 1 ounce) warm water and wash each eye. Never rub the eyes.

Purslane, used in a poultice, helps relieve inflammations. Bruise the herb before placing it in the cloth and lay over the eyes for 15–20 minutes.

A poultice of bruised ivy, placed on the eyelids for 15 minutes, helps relieve swelling.

SPOTS IN FRONT OF THE EYES
Spots in front of the eyes indicate congestion in the system. If the spots are black they indicate congestion in the liver. Drink sesame seed tea using 1 teaspoon seeds to 1 cup boiling water, steep 5–10 minutes, strain, and drink 2–3 cups per day. If the spots are white flecks, they indicate that the kidneys are not getting enough water to flush out the toxins. Be sure you are sipping, not gulping, at least three 8-ounce glasses of water a day. See Liver and Spleen section for more information about cleansing congestion.

STYES
Styes may indicate that the liver is congested. When a sty occurs eat no eggs, fish, or chicken. Collect your own urine from the first elimination in the morning and dab onto the sty to help reduce it. Also use the cleansing diet recommended in the Liver section.

SUNBURNED EYES
For sunburned eyes, use grated apple in a poultice and drink lemon juice and water combined.

TIRED EYES
To soothe tired eyes, use a pad of cotton dampened with witch

hazel or rosemary tea and placed over the eyelids for 10–15 minutes. Grated apples in a poultice are also effective.

Feet and Legs

The feet are, without question, the most abused part of the body. They are constantly under stress and pressure from tight shoes, heat and cold, and all physical activity. Corns, calluses, and blisters on the feet should call attention to abuse, but even tired feet affect every organ in the body. Here are some ways of pepping up not only your feet but the entire system. Foot massages stimulate every organ in the body, relieve tension, and help to regulate digestion. The foot massage charts (see Diagrams 6 and 7) show where nerve endings for the various organs are located in the feet. All diseases may be treated by massaging the corresponding area of the foot.

Diagram 6
FOOT
MASSAGE
GUIDE

(1) Pituitary Gland (2) Sinuses and top of head (3) Ears (4) Eyes (5) Neck (6) Thyroid (7) Bronchial tubes (8) Lungs (9) Liver (10) Solar plexus (11) Gall bladder (12) Kidney tubes (13) Heart (14) Pancreas (15) Stomach (16) Kidney (17) Adrenal glands (18) Spleen (19) Small intestine (20) Large intestine (21) Bladder (22) sex glands and organs (23) hip (24) knee (25) shoulder line (26) waist line (27) appendix

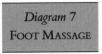

Diagram 7
FOOT MASSAGE

(1) Glands

(2) Kidneys

(3) Shoulder and neck tension

COLD FEET

Cold feet are usually caused by nervousness, which inhibits the circulation. A small amount of cayenne pepper sprinkled onto the soles helps to stimulate the circulation and correct the condition.

CRAMPS IN THE FEET AND LEGS

B-complex vitamins, taken daily, help to ease toe cramps.

The following treatments are helpful for tired muscles in any part of the body.

Leg and foot cramps indicate an improper assimilation of calcium in the system caused by a lack of vitamins D and E. Sipping a glass of warm water and lemon juice nightly helps supply these vitamins.

Raspberry leaves, taken in tea, help soothe cramping muscles and are nutritionally beneficial. Use 1 teaspoon leaves to 1 cup boiling water and steep 5 minutes. Sip slowly 2–3 cups per day as needed.

To massage the legs, elevate the feet and legs and slap the legs as hard as possible with open palms.

FALLEN ARCHES
Mix 1 ounce powdered wormwood and 1 pint pure alcohol (or rum) and allow mixture to stand for 1 week. Shake the bottle each night. After 1 week, strain and rub on the feet morning and evening, and bind the feet with gauze. Continue for 3–4 weeks and take supplements of calcium and vitamin D.

FOOT ODOR
Wash the feet with green soap and soak them in apple cider vinegar water for 10 minutes. Soak the socks in a separate batch of solution and then dry. Repeat daily. Check the diet to be sure sufficient zinc is being supplied.

FROSTBITE
Mullein flowers steeped in oil for several days may be applied to frostbitten extremities to help restore proper circulation.

Your own urine may be applied to frostbitten areas to help facilitate thawing.

GOUT
Gout is a form of arthritis that starts in the big toe. The treatments for this condition are given in the Joints section.

HOT, ITCHY FEET
Soak the feet for 15 minutes in warm water from boiled pota-

toes. Dry feet in a towel with sea salt or dulse powder sprinkled in it, then massage the feet with 2 tablespoons sesame or almond oil.

INGROWN TOENAILS

Ingrown toenails may be caused by wearing shoes that are too tight or by cutting the nails incorrectly. The shoe size should be changed immediately because the nerve endings for various organs in the body may be affected as well as the foot. To prevent ingrown toenails the toenails should be trimmed straight across and not rounded at the corners.

Mix alum with a little water to make a paste and place in a poultice on the ingrown toenail. This will help to draw out the pain and clear the condition. An alum poultice may be used for any type of foot infection.

To prevent ingrown toenails, scratch the top of the nail with an emory board until the toenail is thin. Repeat daily and the nail will grow out flat.

PUNCTURE WOUNDS IN THE FEET

*Puncture wounds from rusty nails and unclean objects should be sterilized and the toxins drawn out with a poultice of pouch tobacco. Mix the tobacco with enough water to make a paste. This poultice will help to draw out the poisons and reduce swelling and soreness. Use a poultice at least for 24 hours, changing several times or until all swelling and soreness is gone. This treatment will help prevent lockjaw and tetanus.

TIRED FEET

Mix 2 tablespoons each camomile, peppermint, oatstraw, red clover, elderberry leaves, linden flowers, fennel, dock, rosehips, and alfalfa in 1 quart cold water. Bring to a boil and simmer for 15 minutes, cool, and soak the feet for 10–15 minutes in the liquid.

VARICOSE VEINS

Varicose veins are caused by excess cholesterol in the system and may be treated with daily lecithin supplements, which help to break down the cholesterol deposits. Drink plenty of liquids to help the system remain clean. The legs may be massaged nightly with a mixture of witch hazel and white willow bark made into a tea. Other helpful treatments may be found in the Heart and Circulatory System section.

Female Issues

Far more than men, women are abused by modern medical philosophies. Thousands of hysterectomies are performed annually and healthy or potentially healthy organs are removed. Even many medical doctors are cringing at the latest trend toward radical mastectomy.

Very little research has gone into finding harmless, natural methods of contraception. Instead, women are taking chemicals manufactured from pregnant mare urine, the consequences of which we will not be certain of for years to come. These chemicals alter the hormonal balance, and women are often unaware that these hormones regulate control of all of the body and not just the ovaries and uterus. Astrological, biorhythmic, lunar, and mental birth control constitute today's

The Handbook of Alternatives to Chemical Medicine   93

limited alternatives, and they, like the chemicals, are not always foolproof. In the coming years, more time and energy will be spent researching alternatives to chemical birth control. But for now, women are advised to use whatever resources are available to them to discover effective, non-chemical birth control methods.

ALL FEMALE PROBLEMS

*Massage the back of the leg behind the ankle to treat all infections or other female problems. Massaging this part of the leg will help to soothe the organs, relax tension, and stimulate proper circulation to the female organs. This area contains nerve endings that correspond to those of the ovaries and female organs (see Diagram 8).

Diagram 8
ANKLE MASSAGE,
FEMALE

BREAST REMEDIES

Vitamin E helps to restore sagging breasts. A healthy diet is also important.

For abscesses of the breasts, use the root and leaves of the pokeroot plant in a poultice. Change the poultice when dry and repeat until abscess is drawn out.

Take 4–5 tablespoons wheat germ daily to help restore sagging breasts caused by nursing, weight gain, or stretched muscles. Improvement should be seen within 3 weeks. Exercises should be taken in conjunction to help strengthen the chest muscles.

Breast cancer or cysts can be treated by using the diets recommended in the Cancer section.

Running sores on the breasts are caused by impurities of the digestive system and blood, or indicate that the bowels are in poor condition. Place a grated potato poultice on the breasts to help draw out the infection, and change when dry. See the Digestion System section for a cleansing diet to accompany this treatment. See also chapter 5, Fasting, for more information.

For caked breasts, steep comfrey roots and leaves in warm water and apply in a poultice to the breasts. Drink the liquid from the steeped herbs and repeat when dry. This will help to soften caked breasts and relieve the soreness and pain.

Menstruation

CRAMPS
*Menstrual cramps have many causes, but usually indicate a lack of calcium and magnesium in the system and a negative frame of mind. Eat fresh, raw parsley or drink parsley tea. This herb helps to warm the body and supply needed vitamins and minerals.

Camomile tea is an excellent remedy for cramps because it soothes stomach tension and relaxes the nerves. Use 1 teaspoon flowers to 1 cup boiling water and sip slowly as often as necessary.

EXCESSIVE FLOW

Shepherd's purse has been known to stop bleeding within 15 minutes because it contains vitamin K. This treatment is excellent for all kinds of hemorrhages. Use 1 teaspoon herb to 1 cup boiling water and steep for several minutes. Take 1 cup as often as needed.

Rushes help to stop excessive bleeding of menstruation. Use 1 teaspoon root and steep 5–10 minutes in 1 cup boiling water. Drink at least 3 cups.

For prolonged menses, press the inside of the leg 5 inches below the knee on both legs at the same time (see Diagram 9). This will help to stop bleeding anywhere in the body within minutes.

Diagram 9
HOW TO STOP
BLEEDING

INCREASING FLOW

Squaw vine is an excellent tea that is good for the uterus and helps increase the menstrual flow. Make a strong tea from the berries and use ¹/₂ cup four times a day.

IRREGULAR CYCLES

Irregularity of the menstrual cycle can be caused by deficiencies of iron or calcium, excessive stress, change in climate or environment, and even diet. A lack of B vitamins, especially B12, can delay menstruation. Here are some teas that assist menstruation. Women who are pregnant should avoid these herbs because they may cause miscarriages. Warning: These herbs are toxic in large quantities. Usage should be discontinued within 24 hours.

Pennyroyal tea helps suppressed menses. Take 1 teaspoon pennyroyal to 1 cup boiling water. Drink $^1/_2$ cup warm tea every 3 hours.

Make a tea using ginger leaves and drink to assist menstruation. Use $^1/_4$ teaspoon leaves to 1 cup boiling water. Honey may be added if necessary. Steep 5 minutes and drink 2 cups.

*Tansy is excellent for promoting menstrual flow. Use 1 ounce tansy to 1 pint boiling water. Steep several minutes, and sip $^1/_2$ cup per day for 2 days.

Sweet basil, taken hot, is good for suppressed menses. Take 1 teaspoon herb to 1 cup boiling water. Drink 1 cup every 3 hours for 2 days.

To assist menstruation, mix $^1/_2$ ounce each black hellborn root, mugwort, wormseed, and valerian. Take 1 pinch of this mixture to 1 cup boiling water and steep for 5 minutes. Take $^1/_2$ cup twice a day for 2 days.

Cottonroot is helpful for bringing on menstruation. Use 2 ounces powdered root to 1 pint boiling water. Drink 1 1/2 cups per day for 2 days.

Birthwort helps induce menstruation and will stimulate delivery of afterbirth. Use 1 teaspoon powdered in 1 small wineglass of white wine. Sip slowly before bedtime. Do not repeat.

Rosemary is well known for promoting menstruation. Use 1 teaspoon herb to 1 cup boiling water and drink 1/2 cup warm tea every 3 hours for 2 days.

Black cohosh, taken 5–6 grains per day, will help to stimulate menstrual flow.

Menopause
Hot flashes indicate that the body lacks hormones. This can be remedied by eating hormone foods daily. Cucumbers, licorice, and sarsaparilla are all high in female hormones.

Passion flower helps to soothe the body during menopause. Use 10–20 drops per day of the liquid extract from the leaves, or if using powder, use 3 grains twice per day.

Pregnancy and Birth
There are many good birthing books on the market, and I heartily recommend home birth. Be sure you check with your naturopathic doctor before and during pregnancy.

*From conception to birthing, raspberry tea should be taken

daily. This herb contains vitamins A, C, B, G, and E, and calcium, phosphorus, iron, and other nutrients that help prevent miscarriages and ease delivery. Use 1 ounce of leaves to 1 pint boiling water and steep for 20 minutes. Drink 10–20 ounces daily throughout pregnancy. Sip slowly.

Squaw vine tea, made 1 ounce herb to 1 pint boiling water, is also helpful to the body for nutritive benefits during pregnancy. Take 2–3 glasses per day.

Pregnant women and nursing mothers should not eat the following foods because they cause gas and colic in the mother and, consequently, the baby: garlic, cauliflower, cabbage, onions, broccoli, and excess quantities of beans.

Cramps in the legs and feet during pregnancy may indicate a deficiency of vitamins B and D. These vitamins should be taken in foods and in supplement form.

During labor, have the mother suck on ice cubes or sip liquids made of peppermint, alfalfa, or raspberry teas. These teas give liquid nourishment to the mother and help to ease tension. Use 1 teaspoon herb to 1 cup boiling water and drink as often as needed. Liquids lost in birthing should be replaced. Drink plenty of liquids, especially if giving birth on a hot day.

INFERTILITY

Infertility occurs when the body does not have sufficient nutrients to support pregnancy. Dolomite (calcium and magnesium) helps to ensure fertility in women. Eat foods that are high in calcium and magnesium or take daily supplements.

MISCARRIAGES

Miscarriages are caused by a lack of amino acids in the system. Drink raspberry leaf tea, rich in vitamins A, B, C, G, and F, and minerals such as calcium, phosphorus, and iron to help prevent miscarriage. Use 1 ounce leaves to 1 pint boiling water and steep for 20 minutes. Sweeten only with honey and drink 10–20 ounces per day. Raspberry leaf tea also helps with an easier delivery.

MORNING SICKNESS

Knotgrass tea helps to strengthen the womb and control nausea. Use 1 teaspoon knotgrass to 1 cup boiling water. Steep 3–5 minutes and sip 1–2 cups per day.

During pregnancy, take fruit or fruit juice first in the morning to cleanse the stomach. One-half hour later, eat bran, barley, or other foods that are high in B-complex vitamins.

Pregnant women should make sure the bowels are clean; this will help to control nausea and protect the fetus against toxins from body wastes. See the Digestive System section for more information.

NURSING

Saw palmetto promotes proper functioning of mammary glands. Take 3–5 berries daily during the last month of pregnancy and while nursing.

Nursing mothers need extra vitamins E and B-complex, and

lecithin. Supplements should be taken daily.

Avocados supply many nutrients needed by the nursing mother. Eat an avocado daily.

*To prepare for nursing, sip a cup of alfalfa tea daily before each feeding to ensure a sufficient supply of milk. This tea also supplies many nutrients.

After a birth, drink plenty of comfrey tea, especially if stitches were made. Comfrey will help repair the episiotomy. Use 1 teaspoon root, leaves, or both to 1 cup boiling water. Steep 5 minutes and take 3–5 cups per day. Use a poultice of comfrey on the incision.

To avoid tearing during birth, the opening to the vagina should be oiled with sesame seed oil daily during pregnancy to promote elasticity. Sesame oil, if rubbed over the entire body daily during pregnancy, will help prevent stretch marks and allow the skin to stretch comfortably.

After the incision has healed, drink pennyroyal tea daily to help draw the uterus and other organs back into place. Use 1 teaspoon pennyroyal to 1 cup boiling water, steep 3 minutes, strain, and drink 2–3 cups per day. Continue for at least 1 week.

VAGINAL INFECTIONS
Vaginal infections indicate that there is an acid-alkaline imbalance in the vagina or uterus. This can result from stress, taking antibiotics, and from birth control methods that change the

balance of hormones. A vitamin B deficiency will promote vaginal infections, and supplements of this vitamin are recommended for all vaginal infections.

To treat thrichomonas and yeast infections, use oatstraw tea to drink, douche with, and bathe in. Drink the tea daily for 1 month to clear up vaginal discharge and strengthen the female organs. Use 1 teaspoon oatstraw to 1 cup boiling water. Make a strong solution of the tea to douche with, and do not repeat for at least 1 week. After douching, lie down for at least $1/2$ hour to allow the female organs to return to their proper place. This also allows the tea to completely saturate the uterus before being allowed to leak out. Oatstraw tea may be reused several times before the nutritional benefits are depleted.

*Vaginal itches and yeast infections respond well to a small poultice of cottage cheese, or farmer's cheese, which is not so wet. Place the poultice on a sanitary napkin and wear daily for 2 weeks. The cottage cheese will stop the itching and draw the infection out of the system. Change the poultice several times a day depending upon the severity of discharge. This remedy is most effective when oatstraw tea is taken daily. Many women say that eating yogurt restores the bacterial balance in the uterus and helps to stop the discharge.

Red sage helps to stop vaginal discharge. Use 1 pint malt vinegar, 1 ounce powdered red sage, and $1/2$ pint cold water. Mix and allow to stand several hours. Take $1/2$ cup several times a day. This mixture works to increase the circulation of the body and strengthen the female organs.

Giant Solomon's seal root is helpful in all female ailments. Make a tea using 1 teaspoon root to 1 cup boiling water, or make into a poultice. Drink 2 cups tea daily in conjunction with a poultice for best results.

Dandelion is an excellent treatment for the female organs. Use 1 teaspoon leaves, roots, or both in 1 cup boiling water. Drink several cups per day. This herb may also be added to salads or soups to give nourishment.

St. John's wort is a good treatment for chronic uterus problems. Use 1 teaspoon powdered in 1 cup boiling water. Drink 3 cups per day for several weeks and then 1 or more cups per week to keep the female organs in tone.

Steep 1 teaspoon each pit root and fennel seed in 1 pint boiling water for 20 minutes to make an excellent douche for inflammation of the vagina or uterus. Use only cooled mixture.

Manzanita is helpful for all female disorders. Do not use if pregnant. Use $^1/_2$ teaspoon herb to 1 cup boiling water. Steep for 5 minutes and strain. Drink 1 or 2 cups per day.

Licorice is a good source of the female hormone estrogen. This hormone helps to build the endocrine glands and is especially helpful in post-hysterectomy care. Use only pure licorice made into a tea or eaten as "candy." Take daily.

Dong quai is the female equivalent of ginseng (which women should not take), and it helps to stimulate the female glands and retard aging. Take about $^1/_2$ teaspoon twice a month.

Blue flag helps stop leukorrhea, which is a white, fluid vaginal discharge. Use 10–20 drops of the juice from fresh leaves to ½ cup water. Take three times a day. When using the powdered herb, use 1 ounce blue flag to 1 pint of water.

Oakbark tea mixed with alum helps to stop leukorrhea discharge. Use 1 teaspoon oakbark, 2 teaspoons alum, and 1 cup boiling water. Sip slowly 1–2 cups per day. Continue as needed.

The female hormone progesterone is contained in sarsaparilla. Progesterone helps the functioning of the ovaries and is necessary for reproduction. Use 1 teaspoon sarsaparilla to 1 cup boiling water to make a tea. Drink 1–3 cups a day as needed.

Glandular System

The glandular system maintains the tone of the body by producing many different hormones and maintaining a balance among them. The glandular system is composed of the thyroid, parathyroid, adrenal, pituitary, and endocrine glands. If there is a malfunction in the glandular system, the body will feel sluggish and run down. To stimulate the system and cleanse it of impurities, massage the spots on the feet that correspond to the glands, as indicated in the Feet and Legs section (Diagrams 6 and 7). If these spots are tender for no external reason, it is an indication that the glands need to be stimulated.

GLAND STIMULANTS AND CLEANSERS
To stimulate the glandular system, eat dark fruit such as grapes and blueberries and drink their juices as well. These

juices and fruits help to build red blood cells and improve the cleansing functions of the glands.

Protein foods help to stimulate the adrenal system. Seeds, nuts, lentils, and beans are good sources of protein.

Cayenne pepper, taken in small amounts of 5–7 grains, will help boost a sluggish system. The pepper may be combined with hot or cold water. Larger quantities will irritate the mucous membranes of the digestive system.

Three to five berries of saw palmetto, taken daily, will help to improve the activity of the glands.

To restore hormonal balances, eliminate all white flours, sugars, and processed foods from the diet. Eat raw, fresh vegetables and plenty of fruit.

Cucumbers will stimulate hormone production. Eat daily in salads or as a snack.

Figs help to feed the hormonal system. For 1 day a week eat only tree-ripened figs and raw vegetable salads made with a lemon and apple juice dressing. This helps to reestablish the body rhythm and supply natural B vitamins.

Combine $1/2$ cup sesame seeds, $1/4$ cup wheat germ, and 3 tablespoons dark honey. Powder the seeds and mix the ingredients together to make small bars. Eat 2–3 small bars daily to stimulate and cleanse the glandular system.

Soy products supply the glandular system with nutrients.

To cleanse the glands, eat nothing but watermelon for 1 day. This diet is especially good during very hot weather.

Yerba mate tea, made with lemon or honey, helps to stimulate the glands and cleanse the system. Use 1 teaspoon yerba mate to 1 cup boiling water, steep 5 minutes, and sip slowly.

Chickweed helps to heal the pineal and pituitary glands by supplying minerals that soothe the system. This herb helps retard aging. Eat in salads or make into a tea using 1 teaspoon chickweed to 1 cup boiling water. Drink 1–2 cups per day.

Valerian helps to eliminate poisons from the glandular system and to stimulate the glands. Use 1 teaspoon to 1 cup boiling water. Steep for 3–5 minutes and take only 1/2 cup per day for 1 week. Wait 1 month and repeat.

Combine 1 tablespoon flaxseed, 2 tablespoons wheat bran, 4 tablespoons rolled oats, and 1 cup vegetable broth and soak overnight. In the morning heat the mixture and sweeten with honey. Eat slowly to help stimulate the proper functioning of the adrenal glands.

Oatstraw tea supplies minerals to the glandular system. Use 1 teaspoon oatstraw to 1 cup boiling water and steep for ¹/₂ hour. The oatstraw may be reused several times. Drink freely instead of water. This tea is especially helpful to replace mineral deficiencies created by exhaustion.

Combine equal parts carrot, celery, and radish juice with 2 tablespoons onion juice. Take 1 cup three times a day to help restore the mineral balance in the system.

Combine $1/2$ glass fresh apple juice, $1/2$ glass berry juice, and 4 tablespoons sesame seed oil. Drink twice a day to supply minerals and nourish the adrenal glands.

Combine 2 ounces rhubarb juice, 1 ounce beet juice, and 1 ounce honey with 5 ounces water. Warm, or drink cold if the stomach is sensitive. Take daily for 1 week to restore energy.

Blend $1/2$ cup soy milk, $1/2$ cup lettuce juice, and $1/2$ cup celery juice together and add 2 tablespoons onion juice. Drink daily for 1 month to supply an energy booster to the body.

Mix $1/2$ cup each soy milk and skim milk with 2 tablespoons brewer's yeast and 1 teaspoon honey. Drink daily to provide energy for the body.

THYROID GLAND

The following conditions may indicate that the thyroid is underfunctioning: feeling cold all the time, low energy, poor growth, and, in extreme cases, an arrhythmic heartbeat.

Dulse is the best thyroid stimulant and should be taken every day to ensure proper functioning of this gland. Use dulse instead of salt in soups, cereals, and whenever liquids are being cooked. Taken daily, $1/2$–1 teaspoon dulse will sufficiently feed the thyroid and help ensure vitality and normal growth.

To stimulate the thyroid, combine 2 ounces Irish moss with 2 quarts cold water and let stand overnight. In the morning bring to a boil and simmer for 10 minutes or until the mixture is reduced to 1 quart liquid. Strain into a glass and take 1 tablespoon each morning for 3 weeks.

Pennyroyal leaves and flowers will help to restore the thyroid system. Make into a tea using 1 teaspoon leaves to 1 cup boiling water, and add honey to give more nutrients. Drink 2–3 cups daily.

Ginger root stimulates the thyroid as well as the parathyroid glands and helps to produce saliva. Use $1/2$ teaspoon freshly grated or $1/4$ teaspoon powder to 1 cup boiling water. Drink $1/2$ cup twice a day.

Bugle will help to reduce enlargement of the thyroid gland. Use 1 ounce bugle to 1 pint boiling water. Drink 3 ounces 5–6 times a day. This helps to improve the appetite.

Mushrooms are helpful for all conditions of the thyroid. Eat in salads or use in cooking.

Headaches

Headaches are caused by congestion in the system, and often it is possible to determine the location of the congestion by the characteristics of the headache. Pressure in the temples and forehead usually indicates that there is tension in the stomach, and throbbing pain often results from congestion in the liver, edie.

spleen, or digestive tract. Migraine headaches are caused by excess starches and sugars in the diet. Foods that are eaten too quickly or washed down with liquids will create gas and putrification in the stomach, which can cause a headache. When an internal organ is congested, it will send signals to the brain that are interpreted as pain in the head rather than pain from the organ. Tension is the most common cause of headaches, whether directly by affecting the brain itself or indirectly by contributing to congestion in the system.

Aspirin is not a good remedy for headache because it cannot relieve the cause of the pain. Aspirin also deteriorates the lining of the stomach and can raise the blood pressure. The best treatment for chronic headaches is a combination of eating well, not drinking with meals, and alleviating stress. This treatment requires a little time, of course, but here are some immediate remedies for headache.

HEADACHE NAUSEA

Cut 3–4 slices of fresh cucumber, place in a bowl with 1 tablespoon dried seaweed, and add enough water to cover. Let the mixture stand overnight, and drink the liquid first thing in the morning. This will help to remove the obstructions in the system that create nausea and headaches.

HEADACHE PAIN

*Combine $1/2$ teaspoon fresh lemon juice and 8 ounces water, as warm as you can drink comfortably. Add 1 teaspoon baking soda and drink quickly while the mixture is still bubbling. In a few minutes you will burp to expel the excess gas. Repeat every 15 minutes until the pain is gone.

The Handbook of Alternatives to Chemical Medicine   109

For pain of headaches and to increase circulation, combine 4 parts dried rosemary, 1 part freshly ground ginger, and 2 parts honey. Make a tea using $1/2$ cup of this mixture to 6 cups boiling water. Steep for 5 minutes, strain, and drink 3 cups per day.

To help relieve headache pain, use 1 teaspoon goldenseal, $1/4$ teaspoon dandelion root, and $1/4$ teaspoon mandrake root in 1 pint boiling water. Steep $1/2$ hour, strain, and drink $1/2$ cup 30 minutes before each meal.

The fresh juice of ground ivy, sniffed up the nostrils, will help relieve headaches.

Basswood helps to stop headache pain. Use 1 teaspoon basswood to 1 cup boiling water, and take $1/2$ cup four times a day.

MIGRAINE HEADACHES

Migraine headaches are a direct result of improper diet. Consumption of devitalized foods makes it difficult for the body to eliminate wastes efficiently. Consequently, the uneliminated wastes accumulate and block the system, making it difficult for the liver to function properly. Pancakes, waffles, pastries, and other gluten foods are particularly difficult to digest. A 3-day cleansing fast and a subsequent diet of raw vegetables and other nutritious foods will bring relief from migraine headaches and help to prevent their recurrence.

Heart and Circulatory System

The heart is one the hardest working parts of the body. Yet, as long as it functions properly, we give it little attention. Vitamins B, C, and E, and dolomite help to strengthen the heart, and proper exercise is vitally important. The heart functions properly if the veins and arteries of the circulatory system are kept strong and supple, and the blood is pure.

CARE OF THE HEART
Blend the following ingredients together and drink 2 ounces one hour before each meal to help feed and strengthen the heart muscles and the circulatory system:

¹/₂ cup tomato juice
¹/₂ cup lemon or orange juice
1 tablespoon brewer's yeast
6 tablespoons wheat germ oil

Pour 1 quart boiling water over 1 cup fresh parsley and allow to steep for 15 minutes. Strain and refrigerate. Drink 3 cups per day as a tonic for the heart.

Angelica will relax the heart and build resistance to infections. Use ¹/₂ teaspoon root powder to 1 cup boiling water. Take 2 cups daily.

Ground ivy helps to regulate the heart and cleanse the bloodstream. Take 1 teaspoon in 1 cup boiling water twice per day or the equivalent amount in capsule form.

Mandrake root helps lower high blood pressure and strengthen the heart. Use ¹/₂ teaspoon root to 1 cup boiling water. Steep 3–5 minutes, and drink 3 cups per day.

Take two garlic pearlies (garlic oil in capsules) daily to help protect and strengthen the heart against circulatory diseases.

Rutin, a yellow powder made from ground buckwheat, helps to strengthen the artery walls to prevent strokes and hemorrhaging. It also makes the capillaries more supple. Take 300–500 mg. daily with vitamin C.

Vitamin E helps reduce hardening of the arteries and aids healthy functioning of the circulatory system. It is found in dandelion leaves, parsley, spinach, mustard greens, turnip leaves, and all green leafy vegetables. Use any of these leaves in a blended mixture to make a good vitamin E drink.

Rosemary helps strengthen the heart. Use 1 teaspoon leaves in 1 cup boiling water, steep for 5 minutes, strain, and drink 3 cups per day. Honey may be added if sweetening is needed.

The adrenal glands manufacture adrenalin and hormones that help tone the blood vessels and the heart. Liver, kidney, wheat germ, green leafy vegetables, soy products, and yeast all stimulate the adrenal glands and the heart.

Pleurisy root is good for soothing tension in the arteries and the heart. Do not use when the skin is cold or the pulse is weak. Use 1 teaspoon root powder in 1 cup boiling water. Take 1 cup three times a day.

Lily of the valley root is good for all heart conditions. Use the plant (not the flowers) for quieting the heart. Use $1/2$ teaspoon root to 1 pint boiling water. Take 1 tablespoon morning and evening. Do not exceed dosage.

*Peppermint tea is recommended to calm the heart and relax tension around the heart. Taken daily, it is said to effectively prevent heart attacks. Use 1 teaspoon herb to 1 cup boiling water and drink freely, at least 1 cup per day.

Taking a small amount of saffron daily helps prevent artery and circulatory problems. Saffron helps rebuild tissue and prevent hardening of the arteries.

White sugar and products containing white sugar are very hard on the heart. Recent studies suggest that excessive ingestion of white sugar may cause heart problems.

Onions and garlic are good for all circulatory diseases. They reduce the possibility of heart attacks and raise the blood's capacity to prevent or dissolve clots. Use onions and garlic boiled, fried, or juiced. Eat approximately 1 clove garlic, $^1/_2$ onion, or both per day.

BLOOD POISONING
Use powdered slippery elm bark and sassafras bark to treat blood poisoning. Put these herbs into a pan with as much water as will be absorbed and make a wet paste. Place the paste in a poultice over the affected area. This treatment is good for poisoning from spiders, insects, snakebite, or other injuries where poison must be drawn out of the wound.

Garlic, taken raw, helps to treat blood poisoning by destroying germs in the system without harming beneficial bacteria. Place a raw lemon over swelling caused by blood poisoning to help draw out inflammation and relieve pain. The juice of the lemon mixed with a glass of warm water and taken internally helps to flush toxins from the system.

CHOLESTEROL AND THE HEART

Excess cholesterol is the result of eating too many processed foods, which leave gluten clogging the system. Lecithin contains phosphorus and aids in dissolving fatty deposits in the tissues and arteries. Take at least 1 teaspoon daily, or take up to 19 grains in capsule form. Some foods that are low in cholesterol are vegetable oil, fish oil, poultry without the skin, nuts, whole grain breads, gelatin, unprocessed cereals, fruits, lean meats, uncreamed cottage cheese, peanut butter, skim milk, sherbet, and all vegetables.

CIRCULATION

Poor circulation indicates a need for vitamins C, E, and rutin. Rutin is ground buckwheat and may be purchased at most drug counters.

To stimulate the circulation, cook the following mixture for 20 minutes or until the texture is mushy. Remove the seeds and eat 1 tablespoon each evening:

1 cup dates
1 cup figs
$^1/_2$ cup corn meal
3 cups water

Two or three grains of cayenne pepper, taken in a capsule or with water, help the circulatory system and help prevent blood clots. Do not exceed dosage.

Bell peppers are good for the blood. Eat one raw bell pepper daily.

Fresh cherry juice helps to strengthen blood vessels and arteries. Drink $1/2$ cup daily for 4 days, skip 4 days, and repeat.

Queen's delight is good for cleansing and purifying the blood. Use $1/8$ ounce powdered root daily in capsules, or mix in fruit juice.

Spicewood bush makes a good tonic for the blood. Break up the limbs into 3-inch pieces and put 2–3 ounces in a double boiler. Pour 1 gallon boiling water over the herb and let the mixture steep for 1 hour. Drink 3–4 cups daily for 1 week.

To help purify the blood, steep 1 tablespoon saffron flowers in 1 cup boiling water for 5 minutes, strain, and place in glass or ceramic container. Take 2 tablespoons 2–3 times a day.

Sarsaparilla is a good blood purifier. Take 1 teaspoon powdered in 1 cup boiling water. Drink 3 cups per day.

Burdock is an excellent blood cleanser. Make a tea using 1 pint boiling water and 2 ounces root. Add 3 pints cold water and boil the mixture down to 2 pints. Strain and drink 3 cups per day. Burdock may be combined with pokeroot, grapefruit, violet leaves, yellow dock, red clover, parsley, or nettles.

Put the following herbs into 2 quarts cold water and boil the mixture down to 1 quart. Take 1–2 tablespoons three times a day to purify the blood:

> *1 tablespoon gentian root*
> *1 tablespoon rhubarb*
> *1 tablespoon sacred bark*
> *1 tablespoon may apple*
> *1 tablespoon yellow dock*
> *4 tablespoons sassafras*
> *4 tablespoons dandelion*

Sassafras is a good blood purifier. Use 1 teaspoon root or bark to 1 cup boiling water, and steep for several minutes. Strain and drink 2–3 cups per day.

Dandelion root or leaves helps build up the blood and eliminate impurities. Use 1 teaspoon root or leaves to 1 cup boiling water and take 2–5 cups per day.

Peaches, eaten daily, help build up the blood and eliminate toxins in the system.

Agrimony helps to purify the blood. Take $1/2$ teaspoon agrimony to 1 cup boiling water. Drink 3 cups per day, or take in capsules.

DISEASES OF THE HEART MUSCLES

Place 1 pound raw unpeeled beets in an earthen jar and cover with $^1/_4$ pound pure honey and $^1/_4$ pound brown sugar. Let the mixture stand for 48 hours and take 1 tablespoon twice a day. This mixture helps to build the blood and strengthen the muscles.

The following 2-day fast will help to relax the nervous system and restore proper functioning of the heart:

On day 1, eat nothing but one kind of fruit all day (apples, peaches, pears, or berries are good). Drink at least 3 glasses of water.

One day 2, eat only brown short-grain rice. Drink at least 3 glasses of water.

On day 3 and thereafter, eliminate all salt and sugar from the diet, continue eating normally.

HEART ATTACKS

Wheat germ is very valuable for cardiac trouble; the d-alpha tocopherol it contains help to prevent blood clots. Take 400–800 IU daily.

Heart attack victims should make a tight fist with the thumb on the outside. Place a hot compress on the chest to help soothe the heart and dissolve clots.

PHLEBITIS

Phlebitis sufferers need to drink plenty of fresh vegetable juices to help dissolve blood clots. Drinking plenty of liquids (especially water) helps to keep the system flushed out. A comfrey poultice on the outside of the affected area helps to dissolve the clot; as does comfrey tea taken internally. This diet should include only fresh juices, raw vegetables, and plenty of roughage such as greens and sprouts. Lecithin also helps to dissolve blood clots and should be taken daily (1 tablespoon). Elevate the affected area for several hours per day.

RAPID HEART (FIBRILLATION)

Rapid heart may be caused by an overactive thyroid gland. This may be the result of excess toxins in the system. Make the fist into a ball with the thumb on the outside and press on the wrist of the left hand to help slow the heart and calm the tension.

The heartbeat may be slowed by placing the hand over the heart and remaining quiet for several minutes. This is the natural inclination of the body after heavy exertion.

Place a compress of hot cloths on the chest to help slow the heart.

VARICOSE VEINS AND ARTERIOSCLEROSIS

Varicose veins and arteriosclerosis result when arteries and veins lose their elasticity and become hardened. Vitamin E taken daily with 2 tablespoons lecithin will, over a period of 2 to 3 years, help soften veins and restore elasticity.

To strengthen capillaries and help reduce rigidity, oatstraw tea is excellent. Use 1 ounce oatstraw to 1 quart boiling water, steep for $1/2$ hour, and drink freely instead of water. Okra also contains the silicon and selenium needed to help the capillaries. Eat fresh when possible, or in soups and stews.

Arteriosclerosis responds favorably to daily supplements of garlic and vitamin E. The garlic will help restore elasticity to the hardened arteries, and the vitamin E will speed up the healing process by supplying adequate oxygen. Eat 1 cup cooked garlic with fresh salads and raw vegetables. Sip plenty of water, but not within 1 hour of eating. Follow this diet for 2 consecutive days per month.

High and Low Blood Pressure

When the circulatory system is tense, the veins and arteries constrict, creating pressure on the blood stream. Thus, tension is the cause of high blood pressure. In turn, the tension is caused by improper diet and stress. Blood pressure may be lowered by eliminating from the diet all fatty meats, spices, salt, alcohol, tobacco, and white sugar. Instead, eat fresh fruits (especially fresh peaches) rolled oats, bell peppers, alfalfa, carrots, celery, parsley, bamboo shoots, zucchini squash, and spinach. All these foods help to lower blood pressure and fortify the blood.

HIGH BLOOD PRESSURE
Raspberry leaf tea helps to relieve high blood pressure. Add 1 ounce leaves to 1 pint boiling water and simmer for 20 minutes. Drink cold, 1 cup per day.

High blood pressure can be lowered by taking 1–3 garlic pearlies and vitamin E supplements daily.

Passion flowers help to control high blood pressure and to

calm nervous conditions. Take 3 grains per day in capsule form or in tea.

*Taking 3–4 alfalfa tablets per day will control both high and low blood pressure and build up resistance to disease. Alfalfa will also help to strengthen the blood cells and arteries.

Asafetida will help to reduce high blood pressure. Use 1 ounce powder mixed with 1 pint boiling water. Take 1 tablespoon cooled liquid per day for adults and smaller amounts for children. Never take more than 1 tablespoon per day. Three grains of asafetida in capsule form may be substituted for the tea.

Cucumber juice or raw, fresh cucumbers help to lower blood pressure. Eat one cucumber daily or drink ¹/₂ cup juice.

Stinging nettles are a good treatment for high blood pressure. Use 1 teaspoon nettles to 1 cup boiling water. Take 4–5 cups per day.

The following diet is recommended for high-blood-pressure patients. In addition to the juices, drink three 8-ounce glasses of water per day. Eat no other foods or liquids during the length of the diet.

On day 1, drink 7 ounces carrot juice, 4 ounces celery juice, 2 ounces parsley juice, and 3 ounces spinach juice.

On day 2, drink 12 ounces carrot juice.

On day 3, drink 9 ounces spinach juice.

On day 4, drink 3 ounces each beet and cucumber juice and 10 ounces carrot juice.

On day 5, drink 3 ounces parsley juice.
On day 6, drink spinach juice all day.

Boil unpeeled potatoes for 15 minutes to produce a liquid that will help to lower blood pressure. Drink 2 cups potato water per day.

Sassafras and prickly ash will make a tea that helps to purify the blood and lower blood pressure. Use ¹/₂ teaspoon each to 1 cup boiling water and take 2 cups per day.

Low Blood Pressure

Excess toxins in the blood are a result of nutritional deficiencies and are the primary cause of low blood pressure. Anemia is caused by poor digestion, iron deficiency, and consumption of devitalized foods. Anemia indicates that the system is not producing enough red corpuscles. Prolonged anemia will rob the bone marrow of corpuscles and will thereby weaken the bone. Low blood pressure and anemia are not the same, but they are related, and the treatments are similar. The symptoms of anemia are unnatural pallor, loss of strength, shortness of breath, headaches, nervousness, cold hands and feet, heart palpitations, and lack of energy. Many of these symptoms are concurrent with those of low blood pressure.

Of course the diet is very important with either condition. Foods that must be eliminated from the diet are white sugar; flours of wheat, oats, rye, and barley; and all starchy foods. Avoid all canned fruits and vegetables, coffee, and non-herbal teas. In addition, eat no animal fats, butter, cream cheese, bacon, pork, duck, or goose, and take only small amounts of honey. Some valuable foods are skim milk, organ meat, muscle meat, tongue, poultry, eggs, and sunflower oil. Eat plenty of brown rice, corn, millet products, rice flour, corn flour and corn meal, fresh vegetables, and fresh and dried fruits. Fresh juices such as apple, grape, carrot, and beet are particularly good. Be sure to include in your diet plenty of B and E vitamin foods as well as those high in calcium, magnesium, and pantothenic acid.

To help raise blood pressure, mix $1/2$ cup soybean powder and $1 1/2$ cups water in a blender at high speed for 3–4 minutes. Strain and drink $1/2$ cup three times a day.

Chives will help to control low blood pressure. Eat at least $1/2$ bunch per day.

Alfalfa is a good treatment for both high and low blood pressure; it helps fortify the blood and build up resistance to disease. Take 3–4 tablets daily.

Vitamin C will help to control the level of blood sugar. Vitamin C also provides long-lasting energy. Take daily in fresh fruits and in supplemental form.

Peas are an especially good treatment for hypoglycemia because they contain vitamins A, B1, B6, and nicotinic acid.

*To build red blood cells, cover 1 pound unpeeled, raw beets with $1/4$ pound each raw honey and brown sugar. Let stand for 48 hours and take 1 tablespoon of the mixture twice a day.

Dandelions contain natural salts which help to purify the blood by destroying acid. Dandelion is an excellent treatment for anemia. Use 1 teaspoon dandelion root or leaves to 1 cup boiling water. Steep for 30 minutes and drink 3 cups per day.

Anemia should be treated with lots of fresh air, good nourishing foods rich in iron and minerals, and by keeping the bowels open. Prunes are an excellent source of energy, contain vitamins A, B$_1$, B$_{12}$, and C, and will promote proper functioning of the bowels.

Treat anemia with tea made from any of these herbs: rosemary, fennel, sage, red poppy, and caraway. Use 1 teaspoon herb to 1 cup boiling water. Steep 5 minutes and drink 2 cups per day.

NOSEBLEEDS

When the blood pressure is high, the blood may break through the tiny capillaries in the nasal cavity, causing nosebleeds. This is one of the body's safety mechanisms to prevent internal bleeding and heart attacks.

To stop a nosebleed, hold the arm on the side of the bleeding high in the air for a few moments to decrease the tension and stop the bleeding. Gently pull on the middle finger on the left or right hand until the knuckle pops. This will help lower the blood pressure (see Diagram 10).

Diagram 10
STOPPING
NOSEBLEEDS

Adder's-tongue is good for nosebleeds. Make a tea using 1 teaspoon herb to 1 cup boiling water and drink 2 cups per day.

Cayenne pepper, taken in tea, helps to improve circulation and reduce blood pressure. Use $1/12$ of 1 grain in 1 cup boiling water and drink 1 cup per day. The cayenne may also be taken in capsule form. Do not exceed dosage.

Insect Bites and Stings

Pure, fresh lemon juice relieves itching from bug bites of all kinds. Rub onto bites. Reapply when needed.

ANTS
Ants will not cross a place where garlic has been rubbed. Take a fresh raw bulb of garlic and rub onto area where ants enter. Repeat when needed.

BEE AND WASP STINGS
Place wet mud on the sting, allow mud to dry, and peel off. The mud draws out the stinger as it dries and helps control swelling.

Honeysuckle juice helps relieve bee stings. Repeat if necessary.

A slice of peeled raw onion placed on the sting will draw out the swelling and lessen the pain.

Wheat germ oil applied to the sting will help reduce swelling and relieve pain. Apply to sting, repeating as often as necessary.

Moisten $1/3$ teaspoon unseasoned meat tenderizer with 1 teaspoon water and apply to insect stings. This helps to relieve the pain and minimize allergic reactions.

Vitamins B and C, taken internally, help the body adjust to stings and bites.

Bicarbonate of soda mixed with water soothes bee stings and reduces swelling.

Basil leaves mixed with water and applied to bee or wasp stings will help to draw out the poison.

Vinegar, dabbed onto insect bites, helps to reduce pain.

EAR MITES
One drop warmed Campho-Phenique in each ear is a good treatment for ear mites. After 1 week use a small amount (3–5 drops) hydrogen peroxide in affected ear and allow to drain. The mites will come out with the liquid.

FLEAS AND FLIES
Rue helps repel flies. Make into a strong tea using 1 teaspoon

herb to 1 cup boiling water, steep for 10–15 minutes, and spray in the room or onto plants.

Put bay leaves in containers of grains and flours to keep out insects.

Place orange peels and cloves in a ventilated closet bag to repel moths.

Make a tea using 1 teaspoon thyme to 1 cup boiling water and spray around windows to repel flies.

Winter savory stuffed into a pillow and placed in the sleeping quarters or into the bed will drive away flies. Camomile flowers may be added for a more pleasing scent.

Pennyroyal, eucalyptus, rosemary, and mint all help to disperse fleas and flies. They may be used separately or together by hanging the herbs in the room or by putting in pillows.

Hips of sassafras placed in a bowl of fresh fruit will eliminate fruit flies or gnats. A strong tea of sassafras sprinkled around the house will keep flies away.

LICE
Cleanse hair with water and green soap, and cut off as much of the "lice hair" as possible. Make an ointment by blending the fruit and leaves of wormwood with lanolin in a blender. Rub ointment onto affected areas to destroy lice.

Larkspur helps destroy parasitic insects. Make a tea of 1 ounce powder or leaves to 1 pint boiling water. Take 10 drops twice a day internally. Use the liquid externally on the hair and repeat 2–3 times daily until condition is cleared.

For lice, make a mixture of 2 tablespoons rue oil, 8 ounces light beer, and 1 quart tobacco water. Apply mixture to affected areas nightly for 5 nights.

Mix 1 quart tobacco water and apply to affected areas daily for 1 week to kill lice.

MOSQUITOES
Rub manzanita leaves or tea onto the body to repel mosquitoes.

Rub eucalyptus oil onto the body or add a small amount to the bath to keep mosquitoes from biting.

Citronella repels mosquitoes. Rub sparingly onto the body. Citronella has a strong scent and may cause allergic reactions.

*Rub powdered sandalwood onto mosquito bites to stop the itching.

A piece of flannel dipped in spirits of camphor and hung in a room will help rid the area of mosquitoes.

SCABIES
Make a solution of 2 tablespoons juniper berries to 1 pint boiling water. Steep for $1/2$ hour. After cooling, divide into 4 parts. Drink 1 part four times a day. Repeat recipe and bathe in the

solution. This treatment will help relieve the itch and drive out the parasites.

Take a bath washing affected parts with green soap to open the burrows of the scabies. Then make an ointment from the ingredients listed below and rub into affected areas thoroughly. Do not change underwear or bathe for 3 or 4 days. Then boil all clothes and bedclothes that have come into contact with the skin.

> *¹/₄ teaspoon zinc sulfate*
> *¹/₄ teaspoon sulfur flowers*
> *¹/₄ teaspoon basillion*
> *¹/₄ teaspoon castor oil*
> *¹/₄ teaspoon gum styrax*

SCORPION, SNAKE, SPIDER, AND INSECT BITES

Rue is an antidote for scorpion, snake, spider, and insect poisoning. Make a tea of leaves using 1 teaspoon to 1 cup boiling water, steep 5 minutes, strain, and drink 2–3 cups as necessary. The strained leaves may be used as a poultice on the affected area.

SNAKEBITE

For snakebite, mix tobacco with saliva or water to form a paste. Apply paste to bite and change when dry. This poultice helps draw poisons from the system.

Avens herb, when worn on the person, helps to ward off snakes.

To keep snakes away from your house, plant onions or members of the onion family nearby.

Use powdered slippery elm bark and sassafras bark to treat blood poisoning. Put these herbs into a pan with as much water as will be absorbed and make a wet paste. Place the paste in a poultice over the affected area. This treatment is good for poisoning from spiders, insects, snakebite, or other injuries where poison must be drawn out of the wound.

Joints
(ARTHRITIS, BURSITIS, AND RHEUMATISM)

The common diseases of arthritis, bursitis, and rheumatism are caused by an over-acid condition and are referred to by various names depending upon their severity and upon which parts of the body are affected. They may all be regarded as "acidosis," and a treatment recommended for one of these diseases will be helpful for any of the others.

Excess acid in the body usually settles in the joints, causing inflammation and pain. In addition, this excess acid inhibits the production of natural cortisone in the body, which feeds the adrenal glands and helps the body metabolize proteins.

The first step toward correcting acidosis is to eat only low-acid or acid-absorbing foods. Eliminate all sugars, white flour products, processed foods that contain chemicals, and high-acid foods such as tomatoes and oranges. Also, avoid salt, vinegar, mustard, pepper, coffee, black teas, tobacco, and alcohol. Potatoes and turnips are among the best foods to eat when suffering from acidosis; they are high in calcium, magnesium, and vitamin D, which help to absorb acids in the system and relieve stiffness in the joints. It is best to build your diet around low-acid foods such as raw salads, fresh sprouts, pecans, brewer's yeast, wheat germ, raw vegetables (particularly potatoes and turnips), and low-acid fruits to help stimulate the digestive system.

ALL ACIDOSIS CONDITIONS

To help restore the acid-alkaline balance in the body, combine the following ingredients and take three times a day, 1 hour before meals:

> *4 ounces tomato juice*
> *1 teaspoon wheat germ*
> *1 teaspoon brewer's yeast*
> *1 teaspoon lecithin*

*Raw potatoes and turnips are excellent for acidosis. Eat as many as possible. Baked or boiled potatoes are also good, but should be eaten without topping (butter, sour cream, salt, etc.). If the potatoes are boiled, use the water as a soaking bath for hands and feet to relieve stiffness in the joints.

Alfalfa helps to relieve pain from acidosis. Eat fresh sprouts daily, take alfalfa tablets, or make alfalfa tea using 1 teaspoon herb to 1 cup boiling water. Drink 2–3 cups daily.

Rosemary, comfrey, or nettle taken in tea, help ease arthritis pain. Use $1/2$ teaspoon powdered herb or leaves to 1 cup boiling water. Steep for 5 minutes and drink 2 cups per day.

Sage is helpful for both arthritis and rheumatism pain. Take 1 ounce (preferably white sage) to 1 $^1/_2$ pints water. Simmer together for 20 minutes and take $^1/_2$ cup when needed.

Cod liver oil helps relax and strengthen the joints when used daily. It also helps reduce popping noises of the joints. Apply externally.

Corn silk tea helps relieve arthritis pain and reduce acidic conditions. Use only fresh corn silk in tea, using 1 teaspoon herb to 1 cup boiling water. Drink when needed.

Parsley tea helps reduce acidosis pain. Use 1 quart boiling water and 1 cup packed parsley. Steep together for 15 minutes, strain, and refrigerate. Use $^1/_2$ cup as needed for pain.

Alehoof (ground ivy) is good for reducing arthritis pain. Use 1 teaspoon to 1 cup boiling water and take 2 cups per day. Crushed ivy leaves may be applied to swollen, painful joints to help relieve those conditions and draw out acids.

A canvas bag filled with oatstraw or with the hay chaff from a horse trough will help relieve stiff limbs when used in the bath. Drinking oatstraw tea (1 teaspoon oatstraw to 1 cup boiling water) helps internally.

Fresh string beans help acidosis because they contain vitamins A, B_1, B_2, and C. Eat daily or drink the bean juice freely.

Jasmine oil helps relieve pain and swelling of the joints due to acidosis.

Cherries and cherry juice help the body eliminate acids and take the bumps out of the knuckles. Take cherries or juice frequently every day for 4 days, stop for 4 days, and repeat.

White grape juice helps absorb the acid in the system. Drink 2–3 glasses daily.

Vitamin C supplements are good for all acidosis conditions. Take 100–1,000 mg. daily when needed.

LINIMENTS FOR STIFF MUSCLES AND JOINTS

For stiff muscles, mix 1 cup vinegar, 1 egg, and 1 cup turpentine and allow the mixture to stand for 2–3 days. Rub the mixture externally into stiff joints or sore muscles.

Wall flower tea is a good treatment for aches of the joints. Use 1 teaspoon wall flower to 1 cup boiling water and drink 1–3 cups daily.

To draw out stiffness from joints and muscles, use orache leaves in a poultice. Change when dry and repeat, if necessary.

Knotgrass juice, when rubbed on broken joints or ruptures, will promote healing. Repeat as necessary.

To soothe aching muscles, combine these ingredients and drink three times a day before meals:

> *$^1/_2$ tablespoon alfalfa powder*
> *1 tablespoon unfiltered honey*
> *1 tablespoon cider vinegar*
> *8 ounces water*

Wintergreen oil rubbed into the affected joints will help relieve stiffness.

For neuritis, the following preparation is recommended. Combine the herbs, take 1–2 tablespoons in 1 cup boiling water, steep for several minutes, and strain. Drink 1 cup cooled mixture ¹/₂ hour before each meal.

1 ounce lavender flowers
1 ounce primrose
1 ounce St. John's wort
1 ounce blessed thistle
1 ounce balm leaves
2 ounces peppermint leaves
3 ounces valerian root

For gout (also see the next section) and rheumatism use birthwort root, which helps cleanse the stomach and lungs of phlegm. Use ¹/₂ ounce powdered root to 1 pint boiling water and drink 2–3 cups per day.

Combine the following ingredients and rub the liniment into affected areas for pain:

¹/₄ teaspoon mustard oil
¹/₄ teaspoon rosemary oil
¹/₄ teaspoon cajeput oil
¹/₂ teaspoon mezeron bark
1 teaspoon capsicum
1 teaspoon wintergreen oil

> *4 teaspoons cottonseed oil*
> *6 ounces turpentine oil*
> *3 ounce gum camphor*

For rheumatoid arthritis, 600 mg. of vitamins C and P (hesperidin) daily help improve the capillary condition.

Thuja, used externally, helps soothe arthritis pain. Boil the leaves and twigs of the thuja plant and use with lard to make a salve. Apply externally when needed.

Combine 1 pound rosemary leaves with 1 1/2 pounds lard and 2 ounces beeswax and place in a large ceramic pot in a hot oven for 3 hours. This process will yield a salve that will help relieve arthritis pain. Strain the salve and apply externally to affected parts.

Lucerne herb, in powdered form, mixed with cider vinegar and honey makes a salve for severe arthritis. Use 1 teaspoon of each in a little water. Also use 1 ounce powder in 1 pint boiling water to make a tea. Steep 5 minutes, strain, and drink 3 cups per day.

GOUT
Gout signals the onset of arthritis and usually begins in the big toe. Corns and calluses that drain the fluid from the joints can contribute to this condition and should be taken care of immediately (see Skin section). In addition, the big toe should be rotated clockwise and counter-clockwise daily in order to help restore circulation.

Plaintain root, powdered or fresh, mixed with lard and spread onto a piece of leather and applied to the toe helps to draw out the acid.

Sarsaparilla, used 1 teaspoon to 1 cup boiling water and steeped for several minutes, helps gout. Take $^1/_2$ cup three times a day for several months or until the condition clears.

Goutweed helps relieve pain in the joints. Use in tea (1 teaspoon to 1 cup boiling water) or as a poultice applied to the affected parts.

Chives are a good food to eat to help reduce acidity in the system and relieve pain. The chives may also be made into a tea and taken daily.

Dandelion tea, which helps circulation, stimulates the red blood cells and helps flush excess acid from the system. Use 1 teaspoon root or leaves in 1 cup boiling water. Steep 5–10 minutes and drink 2–3 cups per day or when needed.

Kidneys and Bladder

The kidneys and bladder are responsible for cleansing wastes from the blood and eliminating them in the form of urine. Without sufficient water, the kidneys become clogged because they cannot excrete these toxins. The residue retained in the body can cause lower back pain and inflammation of the kidneys. Foods containing vitamins A, B2, B6, C, E, and K will help prevent and fight diseases of the kidneys and bladder. Spinach, mangoes, nutmeg, pumpkin seeds, cucumber juice, asparagus, dandelion, grape juice, beets, carrot juice, radishes, and soy lecithin are good sources of these essential vitamins. These foods will feed the bladder and help to prevent formation of bladder and kidney stones.

BEDWETTING

One teaspoon pure unfiltered honey at bedtime helps the body to retain water and promotes sound sleep.

Plaintain, St. John's wort, corn silk, fennel seeds, buchu, and milkweed are all herbs that help prevent bedwetting. Use any one of these herbs to make a tea using 1 teaspoon herb to 1 cup boiling water. Steep 5 minutes, strain, and sip slowly just before bedtime.

KIDNEY AND BLADDER INFECTIONS

*Use dry curd cottage cheese in a poultice over the crotch area to help stop stinging and burning of kidney infections and draw out the inflammation. Use about 1 teaspoon cottage cheese and change the poultice 3–4 times per day. Wear day and night for 2 weeks or as long as needed. Throughout this treatment, drink 5 or more cups of comfrey or oatstraw tea per day.

Flaxseed helps to fight kidney and bladder infections. Use 3 teaspoons seeds in 2 cups boiling water, steep 5 minutes, and drink 2 cups every day for at least 1 week. If you wish to gain weight, eat the flaxseeds. If not, strain before drinking. A comfrey poultice, placed over the kidney or bladder area, will help promote recovery.

All kidney and bladder infections should be treated by massaging between the third and fourth toes. This stimulates the flow of fresh blood to the organs and promotes cleansing (see Diagram 6, page 89).

Juniper berries are an excellent treatment for all kidney conditions. Use several berries in 1 cup boiling water and drink 3–4 cups per day.

Buchu leaves help clear kidney and bladder infections. Steep 1 teaspoon leaves in 1 cup boiling water for $^1/_2$ hour. Use 1–2 cups cooled tea per day. Chewing the leaves and blossoms also will help fight infections.

Vitamins C and E are necessary for proper functioning of the kidneys and bladder. A lack of these vitamins will lower natural resistance.

KIDNEY STONES, GALLSTONES, AND GRAVEL

Kidney stones and gallstones are small "balls" formed by excess cholesterol the body has been unable to eliminate. Care should be taken to reduce cholesterol foods from the diet. Eat plenty of raw, fresh vegetables and vegetable juices. Cleavers helps to break up the cholesterol deposits and should be taken daily. Use 1 teaspoon herb to 1 cup boiling water. Steep 10 minutes and drink cooled tea.

Vitamin C, taken daily, will help to break up the cholesterol and dissolve the stones.

Lecithin helps to dissolve cholesterol deposits in the body. Take 1 teaspoon daily in capsule, crystal, or liquid form.

*Take camomile tea daily for 2 weeks to help break up stones and pass them through the urinary tract and out of the body. Make a tea using 1 teaspoon camomile to 1 cup boiling water. Drink 5–7 cups per day. I have seen kidney stones and gall-stones dissolve completely in 1 week with this treatment. One patient had been scheduled for surgery, but by the end of the week surgery was unnecessary.

If stones are of long standing and are painful, lie down on the floor and slowly sip $^1/_2$ cup warm olive oil. The stones will pass through the body quickly. The warm oil helps to open the ducts and allow the passage of the stones or gravel. Repeat up to three times, if necessary.

Dandelion helps to cleanse the gall bladder and dissolve stones. Use 1 teaspoon leaves or root to 1 cup boiling water, or eat raw dandelion in salads.

Pear juice helps cleanse the gall bladder and restore proper functioning. Drink slowly, several cups per day.

Trailing arbutus is a good treatment for gravel and all diseases of the urinary tract. Use 1 teaspoon to 1 cup boiling water and steep for 3–5 minutes. Sip slowly 2–3 cups per day.

To Stimulate Urination
Dandelion used in equal parts with butcher's broom helps to increase urination. Use $^1/_2$ teaspoon each to 1 cup boiling

water. Steep for 5 minutes and drink $1/2$ cups per day.

Cleavers helps to break up the solids in the urine and increase elimination. This herb can also help soothe irritations of the urinary tract. Make into a tea using 1 teaspoon leaves to 1 cup boiling water. Steep for 5 minutes and drink $1/2$ cups per day or more as needed.

Make a tea using 1 teaspoon fresh corn silk to 1 cup boiling water, steep 3–5 minutes, and drink 3 cups per day. This herb helps to increase the flow of urine and soothe urinary tract pain.

Boil together equal parts horseradish and beer. Take 1 cup three times a day to stimulate urination.

Anise, caraway, and sweet fennel all help to increase elimination. Use in tea or add to breads, soups, etc.

Make a strong tea using 1 heaping teaspoon squaw vine to 1 cup boiling water. Steep for 20 minutes, strain, and take $1/2$ cup four times a day for urinary problems.

Manzanita, taken in tea, is helpful for all kidney ailments. Use $1/2$ teaspoon herb to 1 cup boiling water and steep for 10 minutes. Strain and drink 2 cups per day.

For bladder or kidney obstructions and vertigo, make a tea using $1/2$ teaspoon each vervain and dandelion to 1 cup boiling water. Steep for 10 minutes and drink 1–2 cups per day.

Birch bark and leaves help increase the flow of urine. Make a tea using 1 teaspoon bark or leaves to 1 cup boiling water. Steep for 10 minutes and drink 1–2 cups per day.

Juniper berries help soothe irritation of the urinary tract and increase the flow of urine. Use 1 teaspoon berries to 1 cup boiling water. Steep until cool, strain, and drink slowly. Juniper berries give the urine a violet-like smell.

Too Frequent Urination

When too frequent urination is a problem, use mouse-ear leaves. This herb helps soothe the irritation and cleanse the kidneys and bladder. Use 1 handful leaves to 1 pint boiling water, steep 5 minutes, strain, and take $1/2$ cup four times a day. Treatment should continue for 1 month to prevent recurrence. The following herbs may be substituted: marshmallow root, or rocky mountain grape root.

Liver and Spleen

A healthy, well-functioning liver is necessary to the well-being of every part of the body. The liver inspects and when necessary processes assimilated foods and distributes them throughout the body. The liver regulates the balance of water and salt in the system and extracts and stores sugars, fats, and some vitamins. The bile that is produced by the liver is necessary for healthy formation and maintenance of the bones. The liver also helps to control bleeding and is involved in the production of sex hormones. Obviously, an unhealthy liver will have a detrimental effect on every part of the body, but a proper diet will keep this important organ functioning properly. The spleen works with the liver to distribute blood throughout the body. The spleen also forms and stores blood cells and destroys and eliminates unnecessary blood cells through the liver.

LIVER

A sallow complexion indicates that there is congestion in the liver. Loss of appetite, chronic bowel problems, and spots on the hands, arms, and face are other indications that the liver is not functioning properly.

Vitamins B and C are particularly valuable for treating liver malfunctions. Raw carrots, carrot juice, grapes, parsley, limes, wild yams, bell peppers, nuts, parsnips, spinach, and beets are all high in these vitamins and help to cleanse the liver and spleen.

Use the following diet for 5 days to treat all liver conditions. Do not take any other foods or liquids, except water.

On day 1, drink 10 ounces carrot juice, 3 ounces beet juice, and 3 ounces cucumber juice.

On day 2 drink 10 ounces carrot juice and 10 ounces spinach juice.

On day 3, drink 16 ounces carrot juice.

On day 4, drink 2 ounces coconut juice, 3 ounces beet juice, and 11 ounces carrot juice.

On day 5, drink 2 ounces celery juice, 2 ounces parsley juice, and 9 ounces carrot juice.

CIRRHOSIS

Cirrhosis is caused by a buildup of toxins in the body that

break down the filtering system of the liver and impede the production of red blood cells. Alcohol, tobacco, and chemicals, including pollutants from the air, pass through the liver and tax its cleansing mechanisms. The best treatment for this condition is a strict diet designed to give the liver nutrition that is easily assimilated and to help stop the deterioration. Parsnips and all the foods mentioned in this section are helpful.

The following diet, taken in order and repeated until the condition clears will help to restore the natural rhythm to the liver. The causes of the condition — alcohol, tobacco, chemicals, etc. — must be eliminated in order to complete the recovery of the organ. In addition to the juices listed, raw salads may be eaten using lemon juice and olive oil as dressing. Other foods should be avoided, but liquids such as comfrey tea, alfalfa tea, or teas recommended in the Liver section may be used.

On day 1, drink 7 ounces carrot juice, 4 ounces celery juice, 2 ounces parsley juice, and 3 ounces spinach juice.

On day 2, drink 10 ounces carrot juice and 6 ounces spinach juice.

On day 3, drink 10 ounces carrot juice, 3 ounces beet juice, and 3 ounces cucumber juice.

On day 4, drink 8 ounces carrot juice, 5 ounces lettuce juice, and 3 ounces spinach juice.

On day 5, drink 1 pint grapefruit juice.

May apple helps to stimulate the discharge of the bile. Use 1 teaspoon herb to 1 pint boiling water. Steep several minutes and take 1 teaspoon twice a day.

JAUNDICE (HEPATITIS)

Jaundice, commonly called hepatitis, develops when the liver is producing too much bile. This excess bile causes the skin to turn yellow. Infectious hepatitis is contagious, but as a rule a healthy liver will not contract the disease. Hepatitis can also be caused by severe inflammation of the liver due to an imbalance within the organ. This is a very serious condition that must be treated immediately. If ignored, the liver can be permanently damaged. Cleansing the liver regularly will prevent this type of inflammation. If you should contract jaundice, the following treatments are beneficial.

*To treat jaundice when the patient is exhibiting the symptoms or is turning "yellow," combine ¹/₂ cup each tomato juice and sauerkraut juice. Drink the 8 ounces combined juices three times a day and do not eat. Drink plenty of water. Continue daily until all symptoms are gone and the normal pigmentation is restored.

Mix ¹/₂ cup tomato juice and ¹/₂ cup citrus juice with 6 tablespoons wheat germ oil in a blender and drink 1 glass three times per day. Sip the mixture slowly and take 1 hour after each meal. If jaundice is severe, eliminate foods and eat only fresh, raw salads with lemon juice and olive oil dressing.

Agrimony is helpful for liver ailments, including jaundice. Use 1 ounce herb to 1 pint boiling water. Steep 5 minutes, strain, and drink ¹/₂ cup twice a day.

When nausea accompanies jaundice, mix small amounts of powdered goldenseal root with water. Taking this mixture helps to supply nourishment and to control the nausea.

When jaundice is contracted in conjunction with another disease, such as gonorrhea, drink only hot water for the first 3 days. Thereafter, drink boxleaf tea made from boxleaf hedge using 1 ounce leaves to 1 pint water. Take as warm as possible. Slowly sip throughout the day. Continue until condition improves and energy is restored.

Wall flowers help to control jaundice. Make into a tea using 1 teaspoon to 1 cup boiling water. Steep for 3–5 minutes and strain. Drink 4 cups per day.

CLEANSERS
When cleansing the liver the body may itch. This is a reaction from the elimination of excess bile. To help alleviate this condition, drink a glass of water with the juice of $1/2$ lemon in it. Drink this liquid as warm as possible, first thing in the morning.

Drink one 3-ounce glass black cherry juice every third morning for 1 month. Sip the juice at least $1/2$ hour before eating or drinking anything else.

*Parsley, boiled in water, helps clear liver obstructions. Make a tea using 1 teaspoon to 1 cup boiling water. Take 4 cups per day to help dissolve obstructions of the liver.

Carrot juice is an excellent liver cleanser because it stimulates the system to eliminate wastes. If the skin begins to turn yellow while carrot juice is being taken, it indicates that the liver is congested. Continue drinking the carrot juice. In 1–2 days the skin should regain a normal appearance as the liver is cleansed.

Raspberry leaves help clear liver congestion. Use 1 ounce leaves in $^1/_2$ pint boiling water. Simmer for 20 minutes and drink cold. Take 2–3 cups throughout the day. Continue treatment for 3–5 days.

Steep the leaves and stems of the strawberry plant in boiling water for 5–10 minutes. Use 1 ounce leaves to 1 pint boiling water and drink 2–3 glasses per day.

Drink 1 cup raw beet juice first thing in the morning to stimulate and help cleanse the liver. Sip slowly and do not repeat for several days.

Pure apple juice helps to cleanse the liver and is beneficial in all liver conditions. Drink freely.

Dandelion root will help to stimulate and cleanse the liver and reduce swelling of the pancreas and spleen. Toast dandelion root in the oven and grind. Use 1 teaspoon root to 1 cup boiling water. Brew like coffee and sweeten with honey.

Make a tea using 10–20 drops of blue flag juice in $^1/_2$ cup boiling water, or use 1 ounce powdered herb to 1 pint boiling water. This tea will help to cleanse the liver and restore proper functioning. Drink 3 cups per day.

To help rejuvenate the liver, make a tea using 1 teaspoon each dandelion root, angelica, wormwood, and gentain. Simmer the herbs together with 2 cups boiling water and steep for 10 minutes. Add 2 quarts apple juice and 4 ounces freshly squeezed lemon juice. Drink in small portions, about 4 ounces at a time, for 2–3 days. During these days eat only stewed apples or drink pure apple juice. Repeat once a month.

SPLEEN

Combine 4 ounces hawthorne, 2 ounces each balm leaves and red sage, and 1 ounce each cardamom, cinnamon, and saffron. Steep these herbs in 2 quarts cold water for 24 hours. Add 4 ounces honey, strain, and drink 2–3 cups per day. This will help to reduce swelling of the spleen and stimulate production of blood cells.

Dodder is an effective treatment for diseases of the spleen. Use in a tea made with 1 teaspoon dodder to 1 cup boiling water. Steep 3–5 minutes and strain. Drink 3 cups per day.

Ground ivy helps the spleen to function properly. Make a tea using 1 teaspoon ivy to 1 cup boiling water and drink 2 cups per day.

DIABETES

Diabetes is a serious condition caused by the failure of the pancreas to produce sufficient quantities of insulin. This lack of insulin throws the body into shock. It is very dangerous and, if not treated immediately, can be fatal. The diabetic must replenish the system with the necessary nutrients and avoid starches and sugars until the pancreas and spleen can handle their metabolism. Jerusalem artichokes, string beans, almonds, wild yams, and dandelion will help stimulate the production of insulin. These herbs and vegetables contain high concentrations of vitamins B and C. Vitamin C helps to reduce the need for insulin and should be taken in large doses by the diabetic. All soy products will help to restore proper functioning of the pancreas. Diabetes is not an incurable disease, and with proper diet and nutrition, it can be brought under control.

The following diet, followed closely for 5–6 months or longer, will help restore the natural functioning processes of the pancreas and spleen. Other than the juices, eat only raw salads with lemon juice and olive oil dressing and 2 or more glasses of water daily. This diet provides all the necessary nutrients.

On day 1, drink 7 ounces carrot juice, 4 ounces celery juice, 2 ounces parsley juice, and 3 ounces spinach juice.

On day 2, drink 10 ounces carrot juice and 8 ounces spinach juice.

On day 3, drink 7 ounces carrot juice, 5 ounces lettuce juice, and 4 ounces cucumber juice.

On day 4, drink 7 ounces carrot juice, 5 ounces celery juice, 2 ounces endive juice, and 3 ounces parsley juice.

On day 5, drink 9 ounces carrot juice, 5 ounces celery juice, and 2 ounces parsley juice.

On day 6, drink 6 ounces carrot juice, 5 ounces brussels sprout juice, and 5 ounces string bean juice.

On day 7, begin again with day 1 and continue the order.

Bitter root is good for diabetes because it helps to stimulate the pancreas. Use 1 teaspoon root to 1 cup boiling water. Drink 3 cups per day.

Yarrow contains some of the same active ingredients as insulin and, as such, is very beneficial for diabetics. Make a tea using 1 teaspoon flowers to 1 cup boiling water. Drink 4 cups per day for 6 months. Eat three Jerusalem artichokes per day in conjunction with the yarrow tea.

Huckleberry leaves are a good treatment for diabetes. Steep 1 ounce leaves in 1 quart boiling water for 4 hours. Drink 3 glasses per day.

Dandelion contains many vitamins and minerals and is perhaps the best overall herb for diabetics. Diabetics should eat the fresh greens in salads and drink 3–4 cups of tea daily. Make the tea using 1 teaspoon leaves or root to 1 cup boiling water, and steep for 5 minutes. Strain and sip slowly.

Balm helps to stimulate the liver, kidneys, and spleen and is a good treatment for diabetes. Make a tea using 1 teaspoon leaves to 1 cup boiling water. Drink 2–3 cups per day.

Bananas are particularly good for diabetics because they are easily metabolized and have high nutritional value.

Male Issues

Males need iron, dolomite, and magnesium in large quantities. The predominance of all disorders related to the male organs can be helped by these minerals, plus vitamin E. Pumpkin seeds and cucumbers are high sources of vitamins, minerals, and male hormones. Men should eat up to 1 pound of pumpkin seeds per day or 1–2 cucumbers.

ALL MALE PROBLEMS

Massage the back of the leg behind the ankle to treat all infections or other male problems.

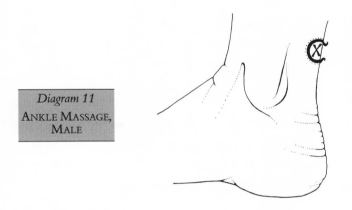

Diagram 11
ANKLE MASSAGE,
MALE

Massaging this part of the leg will help soothe the organs, relax tension, and stimulate proper circulation to the male organs (see Diagram 11).

BRUISED OR SWOLLEN SCROTUM

Bruised scrotum can be relieved by using a comfrey poultice on the scrotum to draw out the inflammation and reduce swelling and soreness. Comfrey tea should be drunk freely. Use 1 teaspoon leaves or root to 1 cup boiling water.

IMPOTENCY

Oatstraw tea supplies silicon and selenium to the system to help restore potency. Use 2 teaspoons herb to 1 cup boiling water and drink freely. Oatstraw may be reused several times and will remain strong.

Calcium and magnesium deficiencies can decrease potency. Supplemental vitamins can help restore potency. The diet must be balanced; any deficiency will impede healthy functioning of the glands.

PROSTATE GLAND DISORDERS

Enlarged prostrate has been successfully treated with magnesium. Take dolomite and vitamin D, three 200-mg. tablets per day.

Urinary disorders of the prostate gland may be treated by soaking 2 tablespoons juniper berries overnight in 1 ounce water. In the morning, add 1 pint boiling water and steep $1/2$ hour. Drink 1 cup morning and evening for 2 days.

*Pumpkin seeds are an effective treatment for disorders of the prostate caused by a lack of male hormones. They are high in phosphorus, iron, vitamins A and B, and calcium and are high in protein and unsaturated fat.

Prostate trouble indicates a lack of male hormones. One or two cucumbers eaten daily will help to feed the glands.

Bruised melilot leaves, made into a poultice with camomile, will help to reduce inflammation of the prostate gland.

Watercress makes an excellent poultice for the prostate. Use to decrease inflammation of the gland.

Vitamin E energizes and lubricates the male sex glands. Vitamin E is found in wheat germ, unhulled breads, green leafy vegetables, cucumbers, pumpkin seeds, peas, beets, nuts, and egg yolks.

STERILITY
Hare lettuce and sow thistle will help restore fertility. Steep 1 ¹/₂ heads hare lettuce in ¹/₂ gallon pure alcohol for 2 days. Take 1 ounce of the mixture three times a day in conjunction with a high hormone diet. Eat plenty of cucumbers and green peppers, which contain calcium and magnesium.

Ginseng stimulates the endocrine system and is a source of male hormones. It should be taken sparingly, approximately ¹/₄ teaspoon once or twice a month. Men who eat beef, pork, lamb, and other red meats do not usually need this further stimulant. Vegetarians, however, may use ginseng effectively. This herb should not be taken by women.

Mouth, Gums, and Teeth

MOUTH
A mixture of goldenseal and myrrh is excellent for trench mouth. Use equal parts of each and massage gums (upper gums down and lower gums up). Also use with warm water to gargle. This mixture also works well for bleeding gums.

Acacia bark is useful for ulcers of the mouth and gums and to help secure loose teeth. Use $^1/_2$ teaspoon bark in 1 cup boiling water, and gargle several times per day.

Arsesmart leaves help to heal ulcers in the mouth. Use 1 ounce leaves to 1 pint boiling water. Drink 1 pint or more of the mixture per day, 3 ounces at a time.

For cankers in the mouth, mix $^1/_2$ teaspoon each barberry bark, bistort, and red raspberry leaves and pour 1 pint boiling water over the mixture. Steep 5–10 minutes and drink often until condition improves.

Gums and Teeth

Your teeth should last a lifetime, and if cared for properly, they will remain strong and healthy. Teeth respond to vitamin C and need calcium long after their formative years. Toothaches and abscesses are signals that there is an obstruction somewhere in the digestive system, and a cleansing diet is recommended. Sometimes the obstruction is due to mucous that does not block the system but may be inhibiting digestion.

Decay Prevention

Strawberries cut in half and rubbed into the teeth and gums help to remove tartar on the teeth and to strengthen and heal gums. Leave the juice on for as long as possible (up to 45 minutes), then rinse the mouth with warm water. Use only fresh strawberries.

Lemon juice and rind help to remove plaque and tartar on the teeth when mixed with the saliva in the mouth. "Chew" the juice to make sure it is thoroughly mixed with the saliva, then swallow slowly. Repeat at least once a week. Scrub the teeth with lemon rind, and make sure all surfaces are treated. The upper gums should be massaged down and the lower gums massaged up. Lime juice or rind may be used instead; both kill bacteria in the mouth when used with warm water.

Alfalfa tablets help to prevent cavities. Take 2 tablets 2–3 times per day.

Lemon juice and flower pumice mixed together should be used once a month to remove any tartar deposits on the teeth. Parsley tonic helps strengthen the teeth. Use 1 quart boiling water poured over 1 cup packed parsley. Steep 15 minutes and strain. Refrigerate the mixture and drink 3 cups per day.

Barley is excellent for all diseases of the teeth and gums. Use in soups or stews.

Witch hazel is a good mouthwash, but should not be swallowed.

The powdered root of water dock is valuable for cleansing the mouth. Use 1 ounce herb to 1 pint boiling water, and steep for 5 minutes. Rinse mouth twice a day.

Powdered dock is a good dentrifice and may be used instead of toothpaste.

Red sage is a cleansing gargle. Mix 1 pint malt vinegar, 1

ounce red sage leaves, and $^1/_2$ pint cold water. Gargle $^1/_2$ cup twice a day.

TEETHING

*Rubbing the gums with olive oil helps relieve soreness and lubricates the digestive system.

Teething babies can be helped through this painful period with camomile tea. Use $^1/_2$ teaspoon camomile to 1 cup boiling water. Steep 3–4 minutes, strain, and sweeten with honey. Test for temperature and give the baby 2–3 teaspoons several times a day as needed.

TOOTHACHE

Aloe vera helps soothe toothache pain. Use juice of plant on gums and repeat often.

Cloves help remove toothache pain and may be used in many ways. The oil can be rubbed into the gums, whole cloves may be sucked for their juices, or the cloves may be mixed with boiling water to make a tea or gargle.

Chewing prickly ash bark helps to relieve toothache pain.

Mullein flowers, when used in a poultice, help to draw out the pain of toothache. Use flowers and warm water, strain, and use the moist flowers in poultice form on the outside of the mouth.

Egg yolk and honey, mixed together and placed on the skin outside the jaw, help draw out pain from wisdom teeth.

Milk from ripe figs is good for toothache. Squeeze out the juice and rub onto gums around tooth.

*Gentle pressure applied to the sides of the index finger on either hand helps relieve toothache pain and relax the tension caused by pain (see Diagram 12).

Diagram 12
TREATING
TOOTHACHE PAIN

$\mathcal{S}kin$

Skin eruptions usually indicate that one of the elimination processes is not functioning properly. This malfunction could be located in the intestinal tract, the kidney and bladder system, or the glandular system. Skin eruptions can also be caused by external irritations from poison oak, poison ivy, nettles, or parasites. Some naturopathic solutions to specific skin problems are given on the following pages.

Thyroid dysfunctions can cause skin disorders. Take dulse (ground seaweed) daily to treat this condition. Massage the corresponding area of the feet as illustrated in Diagrams 6 and 7 (Feet and Legs section) to stimulate the thyroid.

For all skin disorders, combine 2 ounces red clover, 1 ounce burdock, 1 ounce blue flag, and $^1/_2$ ounce sassafras with 1 pint cold water. Allow the mixture to stand overnight. In the morning, bring the mixture to a boil and simmer slowly for 15–20 minutes. When cool, strain and drink 1 $^1/_2$ ounces three times a day until the condition improves.

Brown rice contains many amino acids and, consequently, is good for all skin conditions.

Violet leaf tea is good for all skin diseases. Use 1 teaspoon leaves to 1 cup boiling water. Drink 3 cups per day.

To help control all skin diseases, drink one quart fresh juice per day.

Comfrey contains allentoin, which helps to clear many skin conditions. Make a tea using 1 teaspoon comfrey leaves or root and 1 cup boiling water, steep for 5 minutes, strain, and drink 3–4 cups per day.

Soapwort aids the healing of skin diseases. The powdered herb mixed with water can be applied externally. Repeat daily as needed.

All skin conditions can be improved by fasting and then eating properly after the body has been cleansed.

ACNE, BLACKHEADS, BLEMISHES, AND PIMPLES
Yarrow root tea is an excellent face wash to help control acne. Use 1 teaspoon root in 1 cup boiling water. Steep 5 minutes, strain, and use cooled mixture several times per day.

*One green pepper, one carrot, and one stalk of celery eaten daily for lunch will help to clear up acne and clean the digestive tract.

Apricots, eaten daily, will help to control acne and pimples.

To help clear acne conditions, make a tea using equal parts queen's delight and bittersweet herb. Use 1 teaspoon combined herbs to 1 cup boiling water. Drink freely during the day.

To help clear up acne, take vitamins A and E, and brewer's yeast daily, and apply peppermint oil to the affected area. Repeat daily for 1 month, using only organic products.

For blackheads and oily skin, mix $^1/_2$ cup nonalkaline soap with $^1/_4$ cup each cornmeal and almond meal. Keep the mixture in a closed container and use once or twice per day when washing the face. Dip a wet sponge or cloth into the mixture and rub the face. Allow the mixture to dry on the skin before rinsing with warm water, then with cool water. Blot the skin dry. This mixture helps to dislodge oil and dust embedded in the skin.

Blackheads and open sores indicate that the bowels are in bad condition. Treat the bowel functions and rub lemon juice on the face each night. Wait until morning to wash the lemon juice from the face.

Pimples and other spots on the face will respond well to a treatment of watercress leaves. Watercress helps prevent vitamin deficiencies that affect the skin. Use the fresh leaves in salads for sources of vitamins A, B1, B2, and C, and iron, magnesium, copper, and a lot of calcium.

For pimples and boils, use the birch tree bark. Make a tea using 1 cup bark in 1 quart of boiling water. Boil mixture for a few minutes, cool, and strain. Drink the mixture throughout the day instead of water. Continue until the condition improves.

Cucumber juice, applied externally, will help to heal skin eruptions. Drinking the juice helps to treat the internal causes of skin diseases.

The roots and leaves of avens, made into a tea or poultice, will help to clear the skin of freckles and eruptions.

Blood blisters indicate that the blood vessels are weak. Take oatstraw and dandelion tea daily to help strengthen the blood vessels and supply oxygen. Use $1/2$ teaspoon each to 1 cup boiling water and drink 3 or more cups per day. Eat fresh okra and plenty of fruits.

ATHLETE'S FOOT AND FUNGUS
For athlete's foot, dab vinegar onto affected areas in the morning and evening and soak the socks in vinegar and let dry before using. Wipe the shoes with vinegar to help kill the fungus.

To help clear athlete's foot and fungus, boil 1 cup clover blossoms with water until mixture thickens. When the pulp has cooled, dab onto the affected part of the dry feet. Repeat nightly until condition improves.

Campho-Phenique powder rubbed into affected area will help to kill fungus infections.

Make a tea using crushed green walnut hulls. Drink freely to help kill fungus anywhere in the body.

Combine equal parts blackberry leaves, marigold flowers, raw currant juice, and elder blossoms to make a paste. Rub this mixture into the skin, let dry, and rub the skin with a closely woven cloth bag filled with oatmeal. This helps to scrub off any loose flakes of skin.

For any foot infection, wash the socks every day with green soap and rinse with vinegar to help kill the bacteria.

For athlete's foot and fungus, crush together 2 teaspoons riboflavin, 3 teaspoons niacin, 2 teaspoons pantothenic acid, and 2 teaspoons brewer's yeast powder and mix with 2 teaspoons sesame seed oil. Apply mixture once a day to the affected area, particularly between the toes and on the nails. Put on a pair of clean socks to keep the mixture on the feet. Scrub the feet once a day to remove skin flakes, and reapply mixture after drying the feet thoroughly. Store remainder of the mixture in the refrigerator and add more sesame oil if the mixture is too thick to apply.

BED SORES AND OLD SORES

Combine catnip, brewer's yeast, and whole wheat bread with 1 tablespoon milk, and boil the mixture to a mush. When cooled, bind the mixture onto the skin with a clean cloth.

Change when dry, replacing the cloth each time with a clean one.

BOILS

*To help draw a boil to a head, apply a poultice of chopped garlic. Repeat until the swelling has been drawn out. Do not lance the boil; this may help spread the infection.

BRUISES AND WOUNDS

Bruising easily indicates that the body may have a need for silicon, vitamin C, or rutin. Oatstraw tea helps to supply silicon, and fresh fruits and fruit juices supply vitamin C. Rutin is found in ground buckwheat and may be purchased at most drug counters.

Mix equal quantities of lard and salt together and apply externally to bruised areas to stimulate circulation and replace damaged cells.

Witch hazel bark and leaves, in poultice form, help to heal bruises. Change the poultice several times a day.

For minor cuts, bruises, and wounds, use the beechdrops plant. Apply externally to the cut, bruise, or wound, to promote healing. Use in poultice form or drink in tea.

For bruises, mix the powdered root of monkshood with egg white and apply to the skin over the affected area.

A poultice of giant Solomon's seal root will help to disperse congealed blood from bruises. This treatment also helps to mend broken bones. Change poultice when dry. Repeat as needed.

Powdered arnica promotes healing of cuts and bruises when sprinkled onto injured area.

Bleeding under the skin may indicate a vitamin P (hesperidin) deficiency. See appendices for lists of foods that contain this vitamin.

Open wounds can be drawn together without stitches by applying comfrey poultices. Change poultices when dry and repeat as needed. Drink comfrey tea in addition to help facilitate healing.

For "proud" flesh (excessive growth of tissue, as in an ulcer), or skin that peels off repeatedly, combine $^1/_2$ ounce each poppy seeds and camomile into a bottle with 1 pint boiling water. Apply externally, 1 teaspoon at a time, several times a day.

Make a paste of equal parts charcoal and whole wheat flour mixed with water or spittle. Use the paste in a poultice on proud flesh. Change the poultice when dry, and continue until condition improves.

BUNIONS, CORNS, AND CALLUSES
Bunions, corns, and calluses are most often caused by ill-fitting shoes. These growths will draw fluid out of the joints and cause stiffness.

Massage corns and calluses with castor oil twice a day. The corns will peel off in layers and leave soft, smooth skin, and the calluses will soften.

Boil sweet gum bark into a strong tea, cool, and use daily on corns to help remove them.

For bunions, use 2 handfuls comfrey root to 1 gallon water, boil together slowly for 30 minutes, let cool, and strain. Soak the feet in this tea for 10–15 minutes, both morning and night.

Apply fresh lemon juice to warts, corns, and bunions daily to draw the hardened skin away. Use a lemon juice poultice during the night, changing when dry.

Warts and corns can be destroyed by external application of sun dew juice. Repeat often until the condition is cleared.

Burns, Sunburns

*The juice of the aloe vera plant will help relieve the pain from burns of all kinds. Apply as often as necessary. This juice also helps stop scarring.

For burns, use a comfrey poultice made with comfrey leaves and vaseline or oil rubbed into the surface of the cloth to keep the poultice from sticking.

The toxic effect of sunburn may be reduced by taking vitamin D. This vitamin is also helpful for sunstroke.

For sunburn pain, make an ointment of plaintain leaves and lanolin. This mixture also helps to keep the skin youthful.

CARBUNCLES

Carbuncles are painful inflammations of the skin that discharge pus. A carrot or lobelia poultice applied to the affected parts helps to draw out the infection. Change the poultice often, or when dry. Repeat until the condition improves. Never open any skin eruption because this may invite further infection.

CHAPPED LIPS AND HANDS

Chapped lips are an indication that the stomach is tense. Peppermint, spearmint, or camomile tea will help to soothe the stomach tension. Use 1 teaspoon herb to 1 cup boiling water and drink freely.

Rub powdered arnica onto chapped lips to soothe them. Arnica will also promote healing of wounds, bruises, and irritation of the nasal passages.

Vitamin E oil and wheat germ oil will help to soothe chapped lips. Repeat application as often as needed.

For chapped hands and frostbite, rub wheat germ oil onto hands to help heal chapping and soreness.

COLD SORES

Cold sores may indicate an over-acidic condition in the body. Eat raw potatoes or baked potatoes without salt, butter, or sour cream.

COMPLEXION CARE, FACE, AND SKIN CLEANSERS

Turnips are good for the complexion. Eaten daily, they will help purify the blood, reduce acidity in the system, and destroy bacteria and toxins in the body.

Dandelion greens are a good skin tonic. They help build skin cells and oxygenate the blood. Eat daily in salads or liquify in blender for a liquid tonic.

Raspberry leaf tea works internally to help clean the body and feed the skin. Drink 1–3 cups per day.

To soften and cleanse the face, mix $\frac{1}{2}$ teaspoon egg yolk and $\frac{1}{2}$ teaspoon sour cream and rub gently into the skin. Let dry for 15 minutes and wash off. For best results, repeat 2–3 times a day.

Parsley makes a good face lotion that will increase circulation and help to bring better color to the skin. This lotion also makes a good rinse for oily skin. Use 1 handful parsley in 1 pint boiling water, steep $\frac{1}{2}$ hour, strain, and wash the face with the mixture several times a day. Use a fresh mixture each day.

For a peaches and cream complexion, use fresh peaches and cream! Mix equal parts and apply to the face. Let dry, splash with warm water, and pat dry. Repeat often. Eat plenty of fresh fruits and vegetables.

Mix dried quince seeds with water using 1 teaspoon seeds to 1 pint warm or cold water. Apply 1 teaspoon liquid to the face and leave on overnight to help tighten the skin.

Brewer's yeast helps to prevent wrinkles in the face. Mix equal quantities of brewer's yeast and yogurt to make a facial. Allow to dry on the skin and splash off with warm water. Use this mixture twice a week.

Aloes and camphor help to improve muscle tone in the body and are also helpful for removing wrinkles. Apply externally.

CONDITIONS OF THE FINGERS AND NAILS
Ring-a-round is an infection that causes the finger to swell and become painful. It looks like a ring that extends at the base of the fingernail around the finger, and indicates toxicity in the body. To relieve the swelling, use a comfrey poultice or bind a piece of fresh lemon onto the finger. Change the poultice when dry and repeat until infection is completely cleared. Fasting is also recommended to clean out the bowels and clear the system of toxins.

Alum is an effective poultice for infected or ingrown nails. Mix with enough water to make a paste and change when dry.

Ragged cuticles may indicate a calcium deficiency. Take calcium and magnesium supplements daily and eat foods that are high sources. (See appendices for lists of foods.)

Bumps on the fingers can be caused by eating different kinds of fruits at the same time. The combinations of acids in the fruit cause the bumps. Eat only one kind of fruit per day.

DANDRUFF
To fight dandruff combine $1/2$ cup apple cider vinegar, 1 cup

mint leaves, and 1 cup water and boil together slowly for 5 minutes. Strain and rub the cooled mixture into the scalp. Repeat with each hair wash.

Eliminate all refined sugar and sugar products from the diet for 1 month and take B-complex vitamins daily to help fight dandruff.

For dandruff and alopecia (hair falling out in patches), mix 1 teaspoon bay leaf oil and 7 ounces almond oil. Paint the bald spots with the mixture daily. Continue as needed.

DIAPER RASH
Rub goldenseal combined with lanolin onto the clean baby to help prevent urine burns and soothe rashes from diaper irritation. Repeat with each changing of the diapers.

ECZEMA
*Dandelion greens are a good treatment for eczema because they help to give oxygen to the blood and build cells. Eat in salads or drink in tea made from the root or leaves. Make the tea using 1 teaspoon herb to 1 cup boiling water and drink 1–3 cups per day.

To treat eczema, use hardboiled eggs. Cut open the egg and heat the yolk over a flame. Rub the drops from the egg yolk onto the affected areas. Repeat as often as necessary to help clear the condition.

Dab vinegar on affected areas to help control eczema. Repeat as needed.

Cucumber juice taken both internally and externally will help to clear eczema and skin eruptions. Take 1 teaspoon daily goldenseal in capsule or powder form to help clear intestinal causes. Goldenseal tea can also be applied to the affected areas daily.

Rhatany helps to reduce the discharge from the skin and to draw tissue together. Use a poultice made of juiced leaves. Change when dry and repeat as needed.

Eating several teaspoons of watercress per day will help to control eczema and aid vision, especially night blindness.

For eczema and all skin conditions, mix $1/2$ ounce sassafras bark, 1 ounce burdock root, 2 ounces clover, and 1 pint boiling water and allow mixture to steep overnight. In the morning, bring to a boil and simmer for 20 minutes. Strain and drink 2 ounces three times a day until the skin is cleared.

For dry skin, eat tree-ripened figs. This fruit, added to the diet, helps to stimulate the digestive glands.

GANGRENE

*To treat gangrene, mix equal parts charcoal and whole wheat flour with enough saliva (or water) to make a paste. If possible, use the spittle from the affected person. Put this paste into a cloth and apply to affected areas. When the poultice dries, replace using a fresh cloth. Burn the used cloths. In addition, drink comfrey tea freely.

Beat fresh parkinson root into a powder and spread onto

leather covered with lard. Lay the leather against the gangrenous area to help bring relief. This treatment is also good for moist ulcers.

HERPES (SHINGLES)
Herpes is a nerve condition that may be caused by a lack of vitamins B, C, and D, and sulfur. Spinach, apricots, and alfalfa are helpful when treating this disease.

Mix powdered pharum phos (a cell salt) with witch hazel and apply to external eruptions. This cell salt may also be taken internally to facilitate recovery.

Add kelp to the diet to help eliminate herpes. Use dulse, taken 1 teaspoon daily, or eat seaweed soup.

HIVES
Hives can be treated by applying a mixture of cream of tartar and water. This paste should be applied often to the red marks.

Drink sassafras tea freely instead of water to help control hives. This tea helps to cleanse the blood and restore normal circulation.

ITCHES
*To help stop itching and promote healing of insect bites, stings, or sores, apply pure lemon juice to the affected areas. Repeat when needed. See Insects Bites and Stings section for further information.

To relieve itching on any part of the body, apply wheat germ oil daily. The itch should cease within 2 weeks.

Boil dock leaves in vinegar until soft and combine with lard to make an ointment which will help to stop itching. Apply to irritated areas when needed.

The fluid extract of grindelia (gum plant) is good for itch and poison ivy. Apply the juice to affected areas. Pansy and violet leaves are also effective when used this way.

LEPROSY
Leprosy can be treated with calamint. Use about 1 teaspoon to 1 cup boiling water, steep several minutes, and strain. Apply externally to the skin and drink several cups per day. Repeat applications often.

POISON IVY, POISON OAK, AND NETTLES
*Make a tea using ¼ teaspoon goldenseal to 1 cup boiling water to drink and 1 teaspoon goldenseal to 1 pint water for washing. Drink the mixture six times a day and wash often. About 20 minutes after the initial treatment, the itching from the poison ivy should stop.

To treat poison ivy and poison oak, boil 1 cup water with four cloves chopped garlic. Let cool and apply mixture with cotton to affected parts. Repeat often. Drinking garlic tea is also helpful.

Use madrone or manzanita leaves in tea, 1 teaspoon herb to 1 cup boiling water. Drink and apply the liquid with cotton to the affected areas to help control poison ivy and poison oak.

For poison ivy and poison oak, boil jewel weed down to a mush or crush the juice from the stems of the plant and place on the affected areas. Repeat when necessary.

Crush sword fern and rub onto affected areas to help relieve pain and itching from nettle stings.

Apply wet clay to nettle stings and let dry. The clay will help to draw out the sting and reduce the swelling. Repeat when dry.

PSORIASIS
Dab garlic oil onto the affected parts of the body with cotton to help clear up psoriasis. Repeat daily.

For psoriasis, steep 1 teaspoon sarsaparilla root in 1 cup boiling water for 15 minutes and rub onto affected areas. Repeat as often as possible.

ROUGH, DRY, OILY, CLAMMY, AND SWEATY SKIN
Rough skin may be caused by a lack of pantothenic acid in the system. This acid is found in royal jelly, honey, egg yolks, broccoli, brewer's yeast, and almost all vegetables. Eat plenty of these foods daily.

Fennel tea is a good treatment for clammy skin. Use 1 teaspoon fennel to 1 cup boiling water and drink freely.

For sore, reddened hands, rub on pure lemon juice, rinse, and let dry, or mix together coconut oil, olive oil, and petroleum jelly and apply to hands. Repeat several times a day.

To treat dry skin on the face, press gently as indicated in Diagram 13, in the order of the numbered arrows. Repeat daily. This process helps to stimulate the natural production of facial oils.

Diagram 13
TREATING
DRY SKIN

Dry hands and feet usually result from gulping water and other liquids instead of sipping them. This condition may also be caused by not drinking enough liquids.

For dry, hard, scaly skin, make a tea using 1 teaspoon burdock or sunflower seeds and 1 cup boiling water. When mixture has cooled, rub into the skin several times daily until the condition clears.

For cold hands or feet, use 1 ounce prickly ash to 1 quart boiling water and steep for 15 minutes. Drink 3–4 cups per day to help stimulate the circulation and warm the body.

For sweaty feet, place the feet into water as hot as you can stand it with 1 tablespoon chlorine bleach every night and morning for about 15 minutes.

Oily skin is sometimes a result of a vitamin B6 deficiency. This lack of B vitamins can also cause stiffness in the joints.

RUNNING SORES
Combine black currant leaves, honeysuckle leaves, horehound, and giant hyssop in equal parts and make into a tea. Apply 1 drop of the liquid externally to help heal running sores. Repeat daily.

SKIN CANCER
Castor oil or comfrey, applied in an external poultice, will help to draw out cancerous tissue. Change the poultice when dry. As part of the same treatment, drink 5–6 cups comfrey tea per day. See the Cancer section for additional information.

Goldenseal root, made into a tea and used as a wash, is helpful for all diseases of the skin.

To remove skin growths, use the herb cancerillo to help destroy excess cells. Use 1 teaspoon herb to 1 cup boiling water and drink 1–3 cups per day.

A poultice made of burdock leaves will help to heal skin rashes and ulcerous blemishes. Change the poultice when dry and repeat as needed.

To help remove growth on any part of the body, steep 1 ounce red clover, 1 ounce burdock, 2 ounces Oregon grape leaves, and $1/2$ ounce bloodroot in 1 pint boiling water. Store in glass container and drink 1 cup four times a day.

Spots on the Skin

White blotches on the arms and legs, gray hair, and cold hands and feet are all indications that the body may be low in pantothenic acid. Eat only raw, natural products and eliminate all sugar and refined products from the diet.

Loss of body pigment, or vitiligo, may be caused by the destruction of the acid covering of the skin. Treat with pure mayonnaise, which is almost totally acid. Dissolve 1 cup mayonnaise in $1/4$ cup boiling water with 500 mg. of PABA and apply to the skin on affected areas. Repeat for several days.

To help get rid of spots and blemishes on the skin, mix powdered monkshood root with egg white and apply to the skin. Repeat several times a day.

Stretch Marks

*After a bath, smooth 1 tablespoon sesame oil over the entire body. This treatment will eventually remove stretch marks caused by weight loss, pregnancy, or scars and help to make the skin soft and young looking. Be sure to cover the entire body each time you apply the oil.

Swelling

*Use watercress, comfrey, or crushed ivy in poultice form to relieve swelling anywhere in the body.

WARTS

Warts on the body may indicate that there is excess lime in the system and that body resistance to infection is low. Camomile tea helps to neutralize the excess lime and should be taken 2–3 times per day. Here are some other methods of treating warts.

For warts on the genitals, use the outside skin of the pineapple and rub onto the affected parts. Repeat morning and evening until the warts are gone.

Apply milkweed "milk" to warts daily to help destroy them.

The inside milk from unripe red figs will help get rid of warts. Apply externally once or twice a day until cleared.

To remove warts, use spittle taken first thing in the morning and dab onto the warts. Repeat daily until the warts disappear.

*Apply vitamin E or wheat germ oil to warts daily to help remove them.

Sundew juice applied externally will help to destroy warts and corns.

Houseleek leaves contain malt that helps to remove warts. Chop the leaves and use 1 teaspoon leaves to 1 cup boiling water. Drink 1 cup per day and apply cooled mixture externally to warts.

Soaking the hands in cooled water that eggs have been boiled in will help to get rid of warts on the hands.

Weight Gain and Loss

Millions of Americans are overweight. As we are affluent, so are we overfed. Carrying around excess pounds puts a strain on the heart and on the digestive system. Before embarking on a weight-loss program, you should check to be sure that the problem is not due to a thyroid condition or other organ malfunction. If it is, then you must work to restore that organ to proper functioning before attempting to lose the weight it has caused you to gain. Once you have ascertained that all the organs are functioning properly, you must examine and correct your diet, exercise program, and mental attitude toward weight loss.

To lose weight, you should eat only nonglue foods and eat only when you are hungry. Each person's eating schedule will be unique, so plan your meals according to your stomach and not according to the clock. Avoid processed foods; they are high in calories and low in nutritive values.

The best diet in the world will not help much if you do not get proper exercise. Plan an exercise program for yourself that will give you the needed movement, but do not plan an elaborate program that will not fit in your schedule and that you will be tempted to drop after a week. Walking 1 extra mile per day will help to take off 1 pound per week! Proper exercise will stimulate the system to eliminate wastes and burn off excess fat. Raw fruits and vegetables and high protein meats such as fish, poultry, and lean red meats will provide energy without putting on fat. Lecithin, a derivative of the soybean, will help to break down fatty cholesterol deposits. Lecithin contains phosphorus, and 1–2 tablespoons per day will help to stimulate the metabolism.

Make up your mind that you are getting slimmer every day. Thinking about the weight that you gain while eating a hot fudge sundae will only make you feel heavier and depressed, and more likely to eat more. The mind controls how you feel about your body and can help you lose weight without changing much of your diet at all. Deciding to lose weight is the key. I have found that I can lose 4 or 5 pounds within a week if I make up my mind to do so. On the other hand, if you do not believe that you have will power to lose weight, you are mentally preparing yourself not to do so.

WEIGHT GAIN

To gain weight, do not eat "fattening" foods because they will only put a strain on the body. Instead, eat good, nourishing foods and foods high in B-complex vitamins to help stimulate the appetite and nourish the system. Barley contains large amounts of B vitamins and should be eaten daily in soups, stews, or other cooked foods.

To improve the appetite, steep together $^1/_2$ cup clover and $^1/_2$ cup boiling water. Add $^1/_2$ teaspoon lemon juice, strain, and take 1 tablespoon 3–6 times a day.

Boil 1 handful dogwood bark in 1 quart water down to 1 pint. Let the mixture stand for 1 hour. Strain and take 1 tablespoon three times a day before meals.

Tightly pack 1 teaspoon each wild cherry bark, red alder bark, and cedar bark in a container and cover with boiling water. Take up to 5 cups per day of this mixture, including 1 just before bedtime.

WEIGHT LOSS

The following foods are "glue" foods and should be avoided if you intend to lose weight. These foods interfere with the pituitary gland and hinder the ability of the hormones to metabolize fats. Glue foods literally stick to your intestinal tract and promote weight gain:

ale	jam
all bakery products	pancakes
beer	pasta
biscuits	potato chips
bread	processed cereal
candy	soft drinks
canned fruit	sweet potatoes
crackers	sweet wines
doughnuts	waffles
french toast	white flour
frozen and canned vegetables	white sugar
ice cream	yams

The following foods are easier to digest and help to support the energy needs of the body without adding fat:

alfalfa sprouts	gelatin
all bean sprouts	lettuce
all fresh fruits	raw vegetables
all seafood	rice flour

all vegetable juices   sea plants
brown rice   steamed vegetables
chicken   turkey
grapefruit   whole grain cereals

Here are some aids to weight loss:

Before a meal, mash two bananas thoroughly and combine with 8 ounces soy or goat milk. Skim milk may be used if soy or goat milk is unavailable. Blend together and drink slowly 1 hour before the meal. At mealtime your appetite will be reduced considerably. Two glasses of this mixture can be used to replace the meal.

Two ounces of grapefruit juice mixed with 1 ounce plain water and sipped slowly $1/2$ to 1 hour before a meal will help to prevent the body from taking on weight.

Cleavers stimulates weight loss. Make the leaves into a tea using 1 ounce cleavers to 1 quart boiling water. Drink 3 or more cups per day. For the first six weeks, very little effect will be noticed, but beginning with the seventh week of treatment, the effects will become noticeable. Cleavers helps the body to metabolize and throw off fatty substances through the urine. To maximize the effects, combine with fennel or seaweed.

Steam chickweed greens and mix with mustard, shepherd's purse, or peppergrass to help weight loss. Eat the chickweed mixture and drink the broth.

Bamboo shoots are helpful in losing excess weight. Eat the tender shoots raw, or soften by boiling for 5–10 minutes.

Yerba mate helps decrease the sensation of hunger and aids digestion while supplying vitamin C to the body. Use 1 teaspoon yerba mate to 1 cup boiling water. Drink 4 cups per day. The inner bark of white ash is effective for weight loss. Steep a heaping teaspoon in 1 cup boiling water for $^1/_2$ hour. Drink 4 ounces daily.

Worms

Almost everyone will have worms at some point. They can easily be picked up from the soil, from foods, and from pets, but getting rid of worms is not very difficult. There are three main ways of checking for worms:

1) Observe your eating habits. If you do have worms, you will tend to eat far more than usual and feel hungry more frequently.

2) Check the feces for worms, but this is not a positive test. Some are very difficult to see; others may be external rather than in the digestive tract.

3) Check the base of the nose. If worms are in the system, there will be a small line extending outward toward the ears on either side of the nostrils. Some worms, such as ringworm, will produce a "ring" on the skin. Usually this ring will appear near the elbow or knee, but worms will lodge anywhere in the body that is warm and moist. Ringworm is actually a fungus, but is included here because the treatment is similar to that of worms.

*Garlic is the most effective remedy for worms of all types. First thing in the morning, chop one clove of garlic and place in a spoon. Fill the spoon the rest of the way with olive or sesame oil and swallow. Do not eat or drink anything until the bowels have moved. Repeat the next day and check the feces. If necessary, repeat the third day.

Mix ½ ounce each of tansy, wormwood, and camomile with 1 pint boiling water. Steep for 5 minutes. Drink ½ cup and wait 2 hours before eating or drinking anything.

The fruit of the wormwood tree helps to expel worms. Mix 2 ounces of bark or 20 grains of pulp with 1 pint boiling water. Boil the mixture down to ½ pint and take 1 tablespoon 1–3 hours before bedtime. Repeat twice the first week, once the second week, and thereafter once a month to remain free of worms.

Eat young, tender bamboo shoots boiled in water for 10 minutes to help expel worms. Eat the shoots twice a day for 1 week.

Pomegranates contain a substance that kills worms in the intestinal tract. The skin of the tree root is the most powerful part. Use ½ teaspoon tree root skin to 1 cup boiling water and steep for 15 minutes. Drink ½ cup twice a day for 3 days.

The papain from papaya seeds is effective for expelling worms. Eat 1 tablespoon or drink 1 cup tea made from the seeds each day.

Crushed green walnut hulls made into a tea are a good

remedy for ringworm and tapeworm. Use ¹/₂ teaspoon hulls to 1 cup boiling water. Drink 2 cups per day.

To rid the body of tapeworms, follow this diet for 8 days: Every waking hour, drink 1 cup tea made from 2 tablespoons each crushed pomegranates and crushed male fern root to 1 quart boiling water. Starting with the second day, take 1 table-spoon castor oil with each cup of tea. In addition, eat 1 handful pumpkin seeds every 3 hours. During this 8-day fast, you may sip beef or chicken broth if you are hungry.

CHAPTER 4

Emergency Procedures

rue emergency situations are rare, but being prepared can turn a nightmare into a momentary discomfort.

ARSENIC POISONING

Ingested arsenic will settle in the eyes and back muscles and may cause muscle spasms, paralysis, or softening of the bones. Take teas of herbs that contain sulfur, such as nettle, dock, fennel, or bullweed. Use 1 teaspoon of any of these herbs in 1 cup boiling water, steep for 3–5 minutes, and drink 3 cups per day. Begin a raw vegetable juice diet of carrot, spinach, celery, parsley, and beet juices to help cleanse the system.

BLEEDING AND HEMORRHAGING

To stop excessive bleeding, make a tea of shepherd's purse. Use 1 teaspoon leaves to 1 cup boiling water, steep for 3–5 minutes, and sip the warm tea slowly. Take 1–3 cups daily or as needed. This tea contains large quantities of vitamins C and

K, which help the blood to clot, sometimes within 15 minutes.

Vitamin C and vitamin P (hesperidin) will help to stop hemorrhages. Take up to 500 mg. per day.

To stop bleeding, gently press both legs on the inside of the leg, 5 inches below the knee (see Diagram 14). Hold this pressure for several minutes or until bleeding stops.

Diagram 14
STOPPING
BLEEDING

CORTISONE

Cortisone treatments create severe deficiencies in the body. Prolonged cortisone treatments may cause softening of the bones and make them break easily. Dessicated liver, bone meal, vitamin C, and alfalfa tablets should be taken daily during the treatment and for several weeks after it has been discontinued. It is recommended that you avoid cortisone entirely. Alternatives to cortisone treatments are listed in the sections dealing with specific diseases.

CRAMPS

Raspberry tea will help to soothe cramping muscles. Use 1 ounce leaves in 1 pint water and simmer for 20 minutes. Drink the liquid and use the pulp as a poultice on the affected area.

FOOD POISONING
Drink ½ cup olive oil slowly to help facilitate removal of the poison in the system. Repeat 6 hours later, if necessary.

Take ½ glass hot water with 1 teaspoon baking soda in it to help relax and calm the system and remove the poison food.

HICCUPS
Dill leaf tea will help to stop hiccups. Use 1 teaspoon dill leaf to 1 cup boiling water. Sip slowly to help equalize the oxygen in the bloodstream and diaphragm.

RADIATION POISONING
Mix 1 teaspoon baking soda, 1 teaspoon salt, and 1 quart water and drink 18 ounces every 2 hours, if the condition is severe. When the symptoms appear in the head, chest, throat, glandular system, or nasal cavity, add ½ teaspoon cream of tartar to the solution. Continue treatment until all symptoms are gone. With each glass of the liquid take 3–5 grains calcium.

SCORPION, SNAKE, SPIDER, AND INSECT BITES
Rue is an antidote for scorpion, snake, spider, and insect poisoning. Make a tea of leaves using 1 teaspoon to 1 cup boiling water, steep 5 minutes, strain, and drink 2-3 cups as necessary. The strained leaves may be used as a poultice on the affected area.

SHOCK
Shock occurs whenever there is a major mental, physical, or emotional disturbance in the system. In shock, the body

produces excess adrenaline to offset the emergency and provide energy for escape. This is a defense mechanism and has provided the energy for people to lift cars or run at incredible speeds in order to save lives. Without this kind of physical exertion, the body must find other ways to eliminate the excess adrenaline and restore normal functioning.

Have the patient breathe fresh, clean air. If you are inside, stand or seat the patient in front of an open window. Massage the feet around the areas corresponding to the pancreas and to the organs or part of the body affected by the shock. (See Diagrams 6 and 7 in the Feet and Legs section.) The wrist snap (see Diagram 15) will stimulate the heart and circulatory system to promote elimination of the excess adrenaline.

Diagram 15

WRIST SNAP
TREATMENT
FOR SHOCK

Edward Bach, a British naturalist, mixed together the herbs star of Bethlehem, rock rose, impatiens, cherry plum, and clematis to make what he calls Rescue Remedy. This mixture is is specifically used for treating shock. It is available at most well-stocked health food stores or can be ordered directly from England (see the appendices). Add 1 drop concentrated mixture to 1 ounce water and, at intervals of 15 minutes to 30 minutes, place a small amount on the tongue. After 1 hour reduce the frequency of usage. The amount will vary from patient to patient and according to the severity of the shock. This remedy is nice to have on hand to give comfort to the patient and to help until further assistance can arrive.

SMOKE INHALATION
Use flaxseed tea to treat excessive smoke inhalation from burning buildings, tear gas, etc. Use 1 teaspoon flaxseed to 1 pint water, bring the mixture to a boil, and steep for 5-10 minutes. Strain and sip slowly. Honey may be used as a sweetener if necessary; it also helps to soothe the membranes of the throat.

Slippery elm bark is also a good treatment for smoke inhalation. Make the powdered bark into a tea or mix with warm water and honey to make a gargle.

SPRAINS, FRACTURES, AND BROKEN BONES
Comfrey (also called knitbone) helps to reduce swelling of sprains and to draw fractured bone fragments back together. Use a poultice of fresh leaves and apply to the affected area. The poultices should be changed several times per day. If fresh

comfrey is not available, the dried leaves may be used. In addition, use 1 teaspoon comfrey leaves to one cup boiling water and drink 2-3 cups per day. This tea will help facilitate healing.

TRICK KNEES

To treat trick knee and popping joints, take bone meal and dolomite. To replace an out-of-place knee, kneel on the other leg and stand slowly. As you stand, the kneecap will be freed and will slip into correct position. This process may be repeated several times. A poultice of comfrey leaves or tea may be used on the knee to ensure proper repair. Make comfrey tea using 1 teaspoon leaves to 1 cup boiling water, and drink 4-5 cups per day for 3 days, then 1-3 cups per day for several weeks.

WHIPLASH

Whiplash results when the neck is subjected to sudden shock or movement that the muscles are too tense to absorb. Neck collars are the worst treatment you can use for whiplash! They do not help the neck to realign, nor do they give the body a chance to help itself work back into place. See a naturopath, osteopath, or chiropractor and have the neck vertebrae realigned. Place a silk scarf or cloth on the neck and wear it. The silk keeps the blood moving and helps to relieve pain and tension in the muscles.

CHAPTER 5

Fasting

asting is an old custom, originating in ancient ritual, designed to promote health. The purpose of a fast is to cleanse the system of undigested residue, to stimulate the organs and glands, and to revitalize the entire system. Fasting does not necessarily mean abstaining from food, but does entail following a specific diet of foods, liquids, or a combination of both. Fasting should never result in dizziness, nausea, or fatigue.

Many popular fasts may be detrimental to your health. A fast consisting of only water is valuable only in specific instances and not for prolonged periods of time. Water contains little nourishment and cannot cleanse the glandular system effectively or expel mucous from the digestive tract. Fasting for the first 10 hours of the day and then eating a heavy meal will drastically alter the metabolism and shock the system.

It is not effective to combine eating with fasting. A fast should be followed for at least 24 hours or should not be attempted. Repeated fasting for 1 or more days a week, for months on end, will cause the stomach to repeatedly shrink and expand and may eventually harm the elasticity of the organ. Fasting for extreme periods of time may deplete vitamin and mineral reserves so badly that the body must metabolize its own bone marrow in order to continue functioning.

If you are mentally and physically prepared, however, fasting can be very beneficial to your health. A fast during an illness, such as a strict juice fast during a cold, can help the system to fight infection and heal wounds. Many of the treatments in this book are fasts.

The length of a fast should be determined by your schedule. Do not attempt to fast when you are particularly busy or under severe mental or physical stress. It is important to remember that your method of ending a fast is just as vital as your method of fasting. At the end of this chapter, I have included some thoughts that will help you to break a fast without discomfort and without destroying the benefits of the fast.

GENERAL FAST

*This fast is cleansing for the entire system. Combine 6 ounces papaya concentrate, 4 ounces prune juice, 4 ounces fresh pineapple juice, and 8 ounces orange juice with 1 quart distilled water. Set aside a second quart of distilled water. Once an hour, or less often if you do not feel thirsty, drink 4 ounces of the mixture and 4 ounces of the distilled water from the second quart. You may use this fast for from 1 day to 1 month. A 3-day fast will cleanse the entire body. This is the only fast I have been able to use without experiencing hunger pains. If you are unused to fasting, this is one of the most pleasant. Be sure all the ingredients are organic and the distilled water is pure. Tap water that has been chlorinated will inhibit the benefits of the fast.

RICE AND FISH FAST

A 10-day diet of nothing but brown rice and fish will cleanse the entire system, rejuvenate the spleen, and remineralize a sluggish body. Use short grain organic brown rice because it is the most nutritious. You may eat any type of fish, and you should try to eat a variety of fish over the 10 days.

TWO-DAY CLEANSING DIET

For 2 days, eat nothing but raw vegetables of all kinds and sip three 8-ounce glasses of distilled water per day. Do not eat or drink anything else. This fast will rid the body of debris in the system and help metabolize the carbohydrates already present. In addition, the fast will stimulate digestive enzymes and tone the intestinal tract.

HOW TO BREAK A FAST

How you stop your fast is very important. The stomach is smaller and the body is clean. If you immediately help yourself to a steak or pizza, you will shock the entire system and destroy the benefits of your days of fasting. Do not immediately eat something that will be hard to digest, or you will probably get sick. Here is a sample diet for breaking a fast:

On day 1, eat one apple and sip slowly a small bowl of fresh vegetable broth or soup. Do not use any salt or spice.

On day 2, repeat the menu for day 1, adding a small portion of mashed potatoes and a glass of sour milk or some yogurt.

On day 3, increase the portions of the foods from day 1, adding a small amount of raw vegetable salad, a small portion of brown rice, and some fresh cottage cheese.

On day 4, start to eat normally. Between-meal snacks should consist of fruit only.

During the 4-day diet, be sure to continue drinking plenty of water and fresh juices.

CHAPTER 6

Pets and Plants

Pets

Most of the remedies recommended for people will also help your animals. Domestic animals such as dogs and cats usually need more variety and nutrients than is found in their food. Herbs and supplemental vitamins may be added to food and drinking water to help restore health.

ARTHRITIS
Animal arthritis is caused by an over-acid condition of the system. Vitamin B is essential for treatment, and meat consumption should be reduced and supplemented with comfrey and flaxseed tea as well as natural foods and grains. Use 1 teaspoon each comfrey and flaxseed to 1 cup boiling water, steep for 10 minutes, cool, and feed to the animal. This tea may be used instead of pure water if the condition is a chronic one.

There are other treatments in the Arthritis section off chapter 3 that can be adapted to animal use.

CANCER AND EXTERNAL GROWTHS

Vitamins A and E help to protect animals against cancer of internal organs. Start by adding small dosages to foods and gradually increase up to 200 IU daily. These vitamins will help the animal's system to be more able to control excess cell growth.

Give garlic pearlies four times a day to help animals throw off cancer. The garlic also keeps the system clean, which aids in restoring balances of vitamins and minerals. A vitamin supplement is recommended, and plenty of fresh water.

CONJUNCTIVITIS

Conjunctivitis can be treated with goat milk or goat milk yogurt. Give the animal $1/2-3/4$ cup per day. Supplemental vitamins can also help this condition, especially vitamin A.

DEHYDRATION

Dehydration constitutes a major emergency for cats and may be lethal if not treated immediately. To check for dehydration, pull the scruff of the neck of the animal. If the skin is slow in moving back into place, your animal is dehydrated. Check immediately for diarrhea and make a pot of comfrey tea. Use 1 teaspoon comfrey to 1 cup boiling water and steep for 5–10 minutes. If the animal will not drink, force feed approximately 1–2 ounces of the cooled tea per hour, depending on body weight. Cats, especially, get depressed if they don't feel well and will curl up and die if they are not given plenty of love and attention. The most common causes of dehydration are worms, intestinal viruses, and obstructions of the intestinal tract.

Kelp is a highly nutritious food that will help to stimulate the animal's system. Soak a little kelp in water overnight. In the morning, add 1 tablespoon to the drinking water. Freshly cooked vegetables, especially carrots, celery, or peas, may be added to the animal's food.

DIARRHEA

Diarrhea, in animals and people, indicates that the body is throwing off poisons from the system. Diarrhea is very dangerous to animals and should be treated promptly and with a great deal of care. Veterinarians can sometimes give intravenous injections of a balanced nutritional supplement that can help to restore proper functioning of the system. Diarrhea in cats, especially kittens, may be caused by too-rich foods, such as horse meat, or by eating too much too quickly.

To treat diarrhea, give 1 teaspoon carob powder in 1 glass of water morning and evening. If the condition is severe, force feed $1/2$–1 glass every 2 hours. This amount varies according to the size of the animal.

Vitamin B helps to restore balance to the upset system. Give brewer's yeast powder or mix with meals to help rebalance the bacteria in the system.

Yogurt helps to replace and restore intestinal bacteria in all infections of the digestive tract.

ECZEMA

To treat eczema on animals, combine 2 tablespoons cottage cheese, 2 tablespoons corn oil, 1 teaspoon wheat germ oil, and 1 garlic pearly and rub onto affected area. Repeat at least once a day. Check the diet carefully; this condition usually indicates some congestion in the digestive tract.

FEVER

Animals run a fever when the body poisons are not being thrown off properly. This is nature's way of preventing toxemia. Give a strong mixture of comfrey tea to help bring down the fever quickly and restore balance to the system. Use 1 teaspoon comfrey leaves or root and 1 cup boiling water. Steep for 10–15 minutes and force feed, if necessary, 3–5 ounces per day. The dosage depends upon the size of the animal. For kittens use 2–3 ounces and for large dogs, 5 or more ounces. Comfrey tea added to the drinking water will also help to build up resistance to disease.

FLEAS, TICKS, AND BUGS

Animal flea collars are filled with a nerve gas and DDT. If wet, broken, or otherwise altered, and sometimes without alteration, these gasses can cause extreme reactions in the animals. Flea collars have been known to cause all the hair around the neck to fall out, to create eye infections, and to cause severe skin burns, and death. If you have a flea collar on your pet, or are thinking about buying one, check carefully for any unusual reactions and remove it immediately if they occur.

A pillow stuffed with pennyroyal, camomile, eucalyptus,

winter savory, rosemary, or mint, or a combination of these herbs, will help to drive fleas away from your pet or its bed. Use in the regular sleeping place of the animal.

Rub rosemary oil into your animal's brush before grooming. This will help to drive the fleas away and leave a nice scent. Use daily during the flea season.

Make a collar of leather or cloth soaked in pennyroyal oil or eucalyptus oil. String with fresh eucalyptus buttons to keep fleas off pets.

GAS
Many animals, especially kittens, are plagued with gas. This is usually caused by unfamiliar foods in the system that are not as readily assimilated as is mother's milk. For gas, comfrey tea is helpful when added to the food or the water bowl. Massaging the paws also helps to relieve gas pains. The Feet and Legs section of chapter 3 contains a diagram of the human foot that can been used as a guide.

INTESTINAL INFECTIONS (VIRUSES)
Yogurt, especially goat milk yogurt, helps to restore the natural bacterial balance in the animal's system and replenish diseased cells. Yogurt is especially important if the animal has been given antibiotics. These drugs destroy beneficial bacteria, and the yogurt helps to replace natural intestinal enzymes.

JAUNDICE
For animal jaundice, give only water and four garlic pearlies

per day. Do not feed because feeding puts more strain on the already overtaxed liver and prolongs the jaundice. Continue for 3–4 days.

LOCKJAW

Lockjaw can be caused by infections from unclean utensils, from bacteria-filled horn cuts that are capped off, or from a goat deciding to scratch the "itch" where its horns used to be. This disease can cause severe illness and death if not treated. The best way to ensure that the toxins will be drawn out is to apply a poultice of tobacco. Make a paste of water and pure tobacco. Put this mixture in the poultice and bind in place. Change the poultice several times a day, and continue until at least 2 days after the infection is gone and health is restored. The poultice cloth should be burned after use and replaced with a new cloth. Do not use cigarette tobacco; it may contain chemical impurities.

Give garlic daily in conjunction with the tobacco treatment to help keep the system clean and to destroy harmful internal bacteria.

MANGE

To treat mange, mix equal parts tar and bacon grease and apply to affected parts. Repeat two-three times per day until the condition clears. Give B-complex vitamins or brewer's yeast tablets daily to help facilitate healing.

PREGNANCY

Animals, like people, need extra nutrition during pregnancy.

Vitamins B, C, and E should be included in the diet as well as rolled oats and cottage cheese several times a week.

Raspberry tea should be given instead of regular drinking water to help ensure an easy birth. Make a tea using 1 teaspoon raspberry leaves to 1 cup boiling water, steep for 5 minutes, and add to fresh drinking water daily. This tea also supplies many vitamins and minerals.

Pennyroyal will help to draw the female organs back into place after birth. Use 1 teaspoon herb to 1 cup boiling water and give instead of, or combined with, drinking water for 5-10 days.

Plants

Most plants need specific treatments that depend upon their variety. This section is meant only as general information to deal with common problems.

BUGS, MOTHS, AND INSECT PESTS

Soak five-fifteen juniper berries overnight in 2 cups water. In the morning, strain the mixture, add 1 quart fresh water to the liquid, and spray onto plants. Repeat after rains or when needed. This spray may be used indoors or out on all kinds of herbs, flowers, and vegetables. Rose bushes are especially happy if sprayed with juniper water. The soaked berries may be dropped around the base of the plants to protect the plant at ground level.

Use tobacco water, fixed the same as the preceding remedy, to prevent bugs from infesting plants.

Spread coffee grounds, sassafras, or even cigarette ashes around plants to keep crawling bugs from them.

A simple collar or paper placed on the ground around the roots of vegetable plants such as tomato plants will prevent cut worms from killing them.

PUNY, DROOPING PLANTS

Castor oil or cod liver oil is a good way to make your unhappy plants perk up again. Just put $1/2$ teaspoon on the earth around the bottom of the stalk. The castor oil sinks into the soil and feeds the roots of the plants. This treatment usually produces results within several hours.

APPENDICES

Use and Source of Elements, Minerals, and Vitamins

ELEMENTS AND MINERALS	USE	SOURCE
CALCIUM	Builds bones and teeth and aids clotting of blood. Helps to prevent hemorrhaging and inflammation and ensures normal muscle and nerve response.	Alfalfa, almonds, asparagus, beans, beets, cabbage, carrots, cauliflower, celery, clams, elderberries, goat cheese, greens, horsetail herb, kohlrabi, lemons, nettle, onions, pumpkin seeds, raspberry leaves, tangerines, turnip tops, turnips, and watercress.
CARBON	Helps build strong bones and stimulates body heat.	All types of eggs, fish, and meat.
CHLORINE	Necessary for normal digestion. Helps activate gastric secretions and enzymes.	Cabbage, celery, cheese, dates, eggs, endive, fish, potatoes, onions, oysters, spinach, and sauerkraut.
COBALT	Controls the regulation of appetite.	Apples, beans of all types, gelatin, leafy vegetables, liver, onions, seafood, and whole cereals.
COPPER	Necessary for the formation of iron and hemoglobin.	Asparagus, beans, bran, kale, leafy vegetables, liver, mushrooms, nuts, peaches, peas, potatoes, red and black currants, seafood, whole grains, and watercress.

FLORINE	Protects and preserves bones.	Beets, cabbage, dairy products, garlic, red wheat, rye, seafoods, spinach, watercress, and whole wheat.
HYDROGEN	Necessary for elimination, perspiration, and salivary processes as well as for growth of blood cells and circulation of blood. Helps to soothe nerves and regulate body temperature.	Cherries, fresh pineapple, grapefruit, grapes, lemons, limes, oranges, peaches, plums, tomatoes, and watermelon.
IODINE	Necessary for thyroid health and gland functions. Needed for normal metabolism.	Almonds, asparagus, beans, bran, broccoli, butter, carrots, celery, chard, cherries, currants, dandelion, dates, egg yolks, figs, garlic, hearts, kale, kidney, liver, mushrooms, oats, onions, oranges, poultry, prunes, raisins, seafood of all kinds, sea plants, spinach, and watercress.
IRON	Necessary for the development of red corpuscles and to carry oxygen to cells.	Alfalfa, almonds, anise, apricots, baked beans, beets and beet greens, calendula, caraway, cauliflower, celery, chard, coconuts, dandelion, dates, egg yolks, fennel, hearts, honey, kale, kidney beans, kidneys, liver, nettle, oranges, parsley, poultry, prunes, pumpkin seeds, raisins, raspberries and raspberry leaves, red and black currants, red clover blossoms, red poppy, rolled oats, rosemary, sage, seafood of all types, and watercress.

ELEMENTS AND MINERALS	USE	SOURCE
LIME	Aids digestion in stomach.	Coconuts, cottage cheese, limes, and soy-beans.
MAGNESIUM	Influences muscles, essential to bone structure and nerves. Activates enzymes needed for digestive processes.	Alfalfa, almonds, bananas, barley, beans, brussels sprouts, carrots, chard, clams, corn, cress, dandelion, dates, elderberries, endive, figs, fish, green cabbage, honey, lemons, nettle, parsnips, peas, potatoes, prunes, raisins, raspberries, and watercress.
MANGANESE	Essential for growth and to aid tissue respiration.	Almonds, bananas, beans, beets, bran, chard, leafy vegetables of all types, peas, and whole grains.
NICKEL	Aids the assimilation of sugars in the system.	All fresh greens, all sea plants, bean sprouts, celery, garlic, green beans, lettuce, onions, radishes, shellfish, and tomatoes.
NITROGEN	Builds muscle tone, repairs and builds muscle tissues.	Beans, crab, dairy products, lentils, lobster, nuts, oatmeal, salmon, shellfish, and wheat germ.

The Handbook of Alternatives to Chemical Medicine

OXYGEN	Necessary to dissolve waste products and stimulate circulation. Feeds and stimulates all body organs.	All fruits and vegetables, with apples containing the highest amounts.
PANTOTHENIC ACID	Essential for the healthy functioning of all organs.	All fresh vegetable juices, broccoli, honey, and peanuts.
PHOSPHORUS	Combines with calcium to help build bones; helps to keep the system alkaline, activate enzymes, and metabolize fatty foods and carbohydrates.	Alfalfa, all soy products, almonds, apples and apple seeds, asparagus, barley, beans, bran, cabbage, caraway, cauliflower, celery, cheese, chickweed, corn, eggs, figs, fish, grapes, horsetail herb, kale, lecithin, lentils, lettuce, liver, milk, peas, pumpkin seeds, raspberries, rye, spinach, sweet flag, tangerines, tomatoes, watercress, and whole wheat.
POTASSIUM	Essential to normal growth, healthy muscles, and nerves.	Alfalfa, bananas, beans, beets, bran, cabbage, carrots, celery, cherries, grapes, green leafy vegetables of all kinds, kale, lemons, lettuce, nuts, olives, parsnips, pomegranates, potatoes, prunes, raisins, spinach, and tangerines.
SODIUM	Protects the tissues when water is lost from the body.	Beef, beets, carrots, celery, chard, cheese, cherries, clams, cress, dandelion, eggs, kelp, milk, olives, oysters, peaches, raisins, spinach, tomatoes, turnips, and wheat germ.

ELEMENTS AND MINERALS	USE	SOURCE
SILICON AND SELENIUM	Necessary for healthy hair, skin, nails, and an aid to the mucous membranes and blood vessels. Useful in exhaustion, impotency, and general mineral deficiencies.	Barley, brewer's yeast, horsetail herb, oats, oatstraw, okra, onions, sesame oil, and wheat germ.
SULFER	Necessary for assimilation of body protein, important for liver and skin cells and for the entire metabolism.	Beans, black and red currants, bran, bullweed, cauliflower, chard, cheese, coltsfoot, eggs, eyebright, fennel, fish, kale, lean meats, turnips, leeks, nettle, nuts, onions, oysters, and spinach.
ZINC	Necessary for normal growth, nerves, and healthy functioning of the heart.	Apples, beans, beets, broccoli, cabbage, cress, dandelion, egg yolks, fish, lentils, liver, milk, nuts, oysters, peas, red lettuce, seeds, spinach, wheat bran, and wheat germ.

VITAMINS	USE	SOURCE
VITAMIN A	Aids vision, promotes growth, and prevents infection.	Butter, cheese, cream, eggs, fruits, green peppers, green and yellow vegetables, Jerusalem artichokes, liver, olives, parsley, red salmon, string beans, tomatoes, wheat, and whole milk.

Vitamin	Function	Sources
VITAMIN B₁ (THIAMINE)	The entire B-complex improves appetite, tones muscles, helps prevent nervous disorders, helps stop muscle cramping, and acts as a general stimulant to the system.	Artichokes, barley, bell peppers, dandelion, peaches, prunes, rosehips, spinach, string beans, and sunflower seeds.
VITAMIN B₂ (RIBOVLAVIN)	Essential to children's growth, helps calm screaming and yelling types of tension, and with the entire B-complex helps improve the appetite, tone the muscles, and help prevent nervous disorders.	Brown rice, fresh string beans, Jerusalem artichokes, kale, parsley, peaches, prunes, rosehips, soybeans, spinach, and watercress.
VITAMIN B₃ (NIACIN)	Helps in excessive tiredness, falling hair, muscle cramps, muscle tone, and as a general stimulant to the system.	Asparagus, fish, garlic, parsley, peas, potatoes, and wheat germ.
VITAMIN B₅ (PANTOTHENIC ACID)	The entire B-complex helps to improve the appetite, tone the muscles, and acts as a general stimulant to the system.	Cabbage, cauliflower, grapefruit, oranges, and strawberries.
VITAMIN B₆	Helps to prevent insomnia, oily skin, dizziness, fatigue, stiffness of joints, trembling of limbs; protects against toxins in the system and helps improve the appetite.	Broccoli, carrots, egg yolks, honey, human milk, lemons, liver, molasses, peanuts, peas, potatoes, rice, royal jelly, tuna, salmon, sardines, soybeans, spinach, and wheat germ.

VITAMINS	USE	SOURCE
VITAMIN B₈	The entire B-complex helps to stimulate the system, improve the appetite, tone the muscles, and help to prevent nervous disorders.	Alfalfa and mint.
VITAMIN B₁₂	Helps to regulate menstruation, improve appetite, tone muscles, and prevent nervous disorders.	Broccoli, cabbage, cauliflower, honey, and yeast.
BIOTIN	With the entire B-complex, helps to improve the appetite, tone the muscles, acts as a general stimulant to the system, and helps to prevent nervous disorders.	Cauliflower, grapefruit, honey, lettuce, and spinach.
FOLIC ACID	Aids digestion and the circulation of blood.	Honey, oranges, parsley, potatoes, and spinach.
INOSITOL	With the entire B-complex, helps to improve the appetite, tone the muscles, acts as a general stimulant, and helps prevent nervous disorders.	Cauliflower, grapefruit, kale, and oranges.

Vitamin	Function	Sources
VITAMIN C	Essential to healthy gums and teeth, acts to prevent scurvy, and is also important to the nerves and for prevention of infections.	All fruits, black currants, black spruce, cabbage, carrots and carrot leaves, cucumbers, dandelion, fresh oranges, garlic, grapefruit, green peppers, hibiscus, honey, Jerusalem artichokes, lemons, nettle, parsley, prunes, raspberry leaves, rosehips, spinach, string beans, tomatoes, violet leaves, and yerba mate.
VITAMIN D	Necessary for proper growth of bones and production of good teeth and vision.	Apricots, butter, cod liver oil, cream, eggs and irradiated foods, fish liver oil, honey, lemon juice, milk (very small amounts), spinach, sunshine, and wheat.
VITAMIN E	Strengthens reproductive faculties, muscle health, heart and circulatory disorders; oxygenates the body and lengthens cell life.	Brown rice, carrots, corn oil, cottonseed oil, cucumbers, honey, kale, leeks, legumes, lemons, lettuce, mustard leaves, nettle, nuts, parsley, pears, potatoes, pumpkin seeds, raspberry leaves, spinach, turnips and turnip leaves, and wheat germ.
VITAMIN F	Required by the blood for coagulation.	Alfalfa, all green vegetables, apples and apple pits, cherries, grapes, olive oil, and orange peels.
VITAMIN G	Regarded as an aid to general health with special importance for the skin. Also important in the coagulation of the blood and the stomach processes.	Alfalfa, brains, cereal, cheese, cranberries, eggs, greens, liver, potatoes, and raspberry leaves.

VITAMINS	USE	SOURCE
VITAMIN K	Essential in the clotting ability of the blood.	Alfalfa, all greens, apple pits, brown rice, cabbage, carrots, parsley, rosehips, shepherd's purse, spinach, and turnips.
VITAMIN P (Hesperidin)	Important to the well-being of every cell in the body, helps coagulation of the blood, capillary action, control of hemorrhaging, and to throw off body wastes.	Alfalfa, apple pits, apricots, blackberries, black currants, carrots, cherries, grapes, lemons, orange peels, plums, rosehips, rutin, spinach, and white grapefruit.

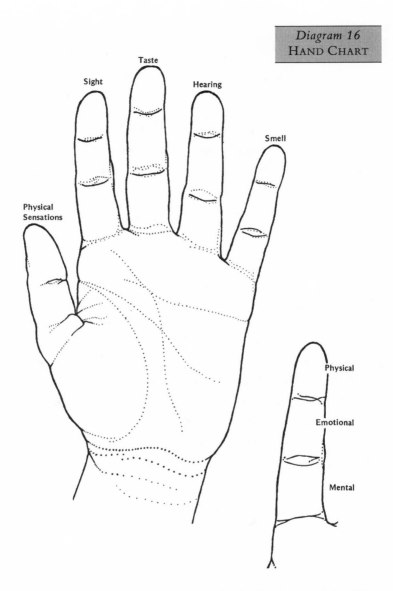

Massaging each finger stimulates a particular sensory capacity. The sections of the fingers represent mental, physical, and emotional influences as indicated. This type of massage may be used to facilitate the healing process.

Herbal Sources

If you are in the market for herbs that your local grocery or health food store doesn't have and you are unable to recognize the ones you need growing wild, there are several excellent herb stores located in different parts of the country. Here is a short list:

INDIANA BOTANIC GARDENS
P.O. Box 5
Hammond, Indiana 46325
(800) 514-1068

The Indiana Botanic Gardens grow and stock thousands of different herbs, seeds, and plants, but buying plants is tricky if you live across state lines. If you need an herb list, almanac, or just want information, they have comprehensive files and will answer you promptly. If the herbs you need are not on their list, write to them anyway, as they have found herbs for me that are listed in their catalog under entirely different names. The Indiana Botanic Gardens grow most of their own herbs and the supply is fresh and fairly inexpensive.

LHASA KARNAK HERB COMPANY
2513 Telegraph Avenue
Berkeley, California 94704
or
1938 Shattuck Avenue
Berkeley, California 94704

Lhasa Karnak stocks herbs, spices, ginseng, and even herbal smoking mixtures and tea strainers. They sell both large and small quantities and will help you find what you need if they don't stock it. Since I live near Lhasa Karnak, I use this supplier often and have been quite happy with the freshness and quality of the herbs, especially imported herbs, the quality of which can vary quite a bit. They have a complete catalog of the products they stock, available for $1.00. It is revised and updated often. When buying from them in person, I have found low prices and broad variety.

MT. ROSE HERBS
20818 High Street
North San Juan, California 95960
(800) 879-3337

Mt. Rose Herbs is a great source for organically grown herbs. They are a supplier for herbalists and maintain a varied supply of dried herbs. They have a catalog available for $1.00. This again is a friendly, knowledgeable source for quality herbs.

BILL'S PHARMACY
33 Van Buren
Eureka Springs, Arkansas 72632

Owned by a registered pharmacist who specializes in over 300 herbs and oils as well as a complete line of homeopathic medicines, vitamins, and supplements. Mail order information is available from the above address. Formerly known as Stamps Apothecary, Bill's Pharmacy is a good source for homeopathic remedies.

NO COMMON SCENTS, INC.
King's Yard
Yellow Springs, Ohio 45387
(800) 686-0012

An excellent wide selection (over 300) of herbs, spices, teas, and botanicals.

Great source for imported spices and teas. They offer low prices, high quality, and quick mail-order response. They also have a free catalog.

THE HERB STOP
414 South Mill Avenue, Suite 113
Tempe, Arizona 85281

The Herb Stop has a wide selection of herbs, homeopathic remedies, Chinese patent formulas, essential oils, flower essences, and ayurvedic products. They also offer herb classes for beginners. Knowledgeable and friendly, they can help you locate rare or hard-to-find herbs.

REFERENCES

The books listed below are by no means the total of those available, but they are books I have used and like.

Edward Bach, *Heal Thyself,* C.W. Daniel Company, Ltd., London, England.

Nicholas Culpeper, *Culpeper's Complete Herbal*, Foulsham and Company, Ltd., New York.

Maud Grieve, *A Modern Herbal*, 2 volumes, Dover Publications, Inc., New York.

Eunice D. Ingham, *Original Stories of Eunice D. Ingham: Stories the Feet Can Tell Thru Reflexology*, Ingham Publishing, Rochester, New York.

Jethro Kloss, *Back to Eden*, Back to Eden Books, Santa Barbara, California.

INDEX

A

B

nausea associated with, 109
Heart and circulatory system, 25,
110–119
Heart
attacks, 117, 123
care of, 111–113
Heartbeat
arrhythmic, 107
rapid (fibrillation), 118
Heartburn. 62, 69–72
Hemorrhaging, 21, 112, 185–186
Hemorrhoids, 72–73
Hepatitis. *See* Jaundice
Herbal treatments, how to prepare,
11–15
Herbs
commercial sources of, 218–220
growing and storing of, 12
Hernias, 15
Herpes, 168
Hiccups, 71, 187
Hives, 168
Hoarseness, 55
Home medicine chest, 15
Hormones, 29
female, 103, 104
male, 74, 149, 150
Hot flashes, 98
Hypochondria, 25
Hypoglycemia, 122
Hysteria, 25

I

Impotency, 150
Indigestion, 4, 5, 62, 67, 71
Infections
bladder, xiii, 136–137
chest, 44, 48, 52, 57
ear, 77–78
eye, 83–84
finger and nail, 165
internal, xiii, 136–137

kidney, xiii, 136–137
poultices for, 13
Infertility, 99–100
Influenza. *See* Flu
Ingrown nails, 165
Insanity, 28
Insect
bites and stings of, 124–129, 168
infestation of plants, 205–206
repellents for, 125–127
Insomnia, xiii, xiv, 21, 28–31
Internal organs, diagram of, viii
Intestinal tract
infections of, in pets, 203
poisoning, 76
toning of, 22
Intestines, 65–72
Itching, 15, 144, 168–169. *See also* Insect
Bites and Stings
of feet, 91–92
of vagina, 102
Jaundice (hepatitis), 143–144
in pets, 203–204
Joint problems, 129–135, 190

K

Kidneys, 5, 19, 135–140
cleansing of, 48
disease of, 38
infections of, xiii, 136–137
stimulator for, 148
stones in, 136, 137
Knees, trick, 190. *See also* Joints

L

Laryngitis, 53, 62
Laxatives, 73–76
Legs, 89–93. *See also* Paralysis
cramps in, 90, 99
varicose veins in, 42, 93, 118

V

Vaginal infections, 101–104
Varicose veins, 42, 93, 118.
  See also Heart and circulatory system
Vegetables, guidelines to eating of, 6
Vertigo, 139
Viruses, in pets, 203
Vision, improving, xiv–xv, 84–85
Vitamins, uses and sources of 212–216
Vitiligo, 173

W

Warts, 162, 174
  genital, 174
Water brash. *See* Burping
Wasp stings, 124–125
Water, importance of drinking. xiii,
  5, 19, 135
Weariness, 23
Weight gain and loss, 175–179.
  See also Overeating
Whiplash, 13, 190
Worms, 179–181
Worry, as cause of disease, 7–8
Wounds, 15, 92, 113, 160–161
  poultices for, 13
Wrinkles, 165

Y

Yeast infections, 102

ABOUT THE AUTHORS

MILDRED JACKSON was a naturopathic doctor practicing in Albany, California. Her varied experiences included work in obesity clinics, convalescent hospitals, with undernourished children, and more than twenty-five years of private practice. She studied both drugless and chemical nursing, took three years of dental schooling and more than 300 courses in various types of healing, including iridiagnosis, color and flower healing, American, European, and Eastern herbalism, and massage. In addition to her private practice, she taught a weekly course in alternative healing.

*

In addition to earning a naturopathy doctorate in Great Britain, TERRI K. TEAGUE also received her doctorate in chiropractic from Life Chiropractic College—West in San Lorenzo, California. She counseled emotionally disturbed adults, taught classes in alternative healing methods at several Bay Area institutions, and was a featured guest author on radio and television talk shows. She completed her undergraduate studies at Lenoir Rhyne College in Hickory, North Carolina, where she received her B.A.

*

Mildred and Terri gave lectures for the Wholistic Health and Nutrition Institute of Mill Valley, California, the Berkeley Holistic Health Center, and retreats sponsored by the California School of Herbal Studies in Guerneville. Their articles have been published in various magazines, such as *Alternatives*, *Well Being*, and *Rain: Journal of Appropriate Technology*.

New World Library is dedicated to
publishing books and cassettes that inspire
and challenge us to improve the quality
of our lives and our world.

Our books and tapes are available
in bookstores everywhere.
For a catalog of our complete library
of fine books and cassettes, contact:

New World Library
14 Pamaron Way
Novato, CA 94949

Phone: (415) 884-2100
Fax: (415) 884-2199
Or call toll free: (800) 972-6657
Catalog requests: Ext. 900
Ordering: Ext. 902

E-mail: escort@nwlib.com
http://www.nwlib.com